High Resolution and High Definition Anorectal Manometry

Massimo Bellini

Editor

High Resolution and High Definition Anorectal Manometry

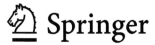 Springer

Editor
Massimo Bellini
Gastrointestinal Unit, Department of Gastroenterology Unit
Department of Translational Research and New Technologies in Medicine and Surgery
University of Pisa
Pisa
Italy

ISBN 978-3-030-32421-6   ISBN 978-3-030-32419-3   (eBook)
https://doi.org/10.1007/978-3-030-32419-3

This Springer imprint is published by the registered company Springer Nature Switzerland AG
The registered company address is: Gewerbestrasse 11, 6330 Cham, Switzerland

Preface

The book provides a comprehensive overview of high-resolution and high-definition anorectal manometry (HRAM/HDAM), showing the possible benefits of a wider use of these techniques in clinical practice, as well as their limitations. Although these techniques provide fresh insights into anorectal function and offer a new perspective on the pathophysiologic mechanisms of many defecation disturbances, there is a need to clarify whether their use has beneficial effects on clinical management compared to conventional manometry. There is still a considerable way to go to gain the clinical diffusion of esophageal HRM, which has become the gold standard in studying esophageal motility. Indeed, many gastroenterologists and surgeons are convinced that further studies are necessary in order to be able to recommend HRAM and HDAM over and above conventional anorectal manometry. The first part of the book presents anorectal anatomy and pathophysiology, highlighting the indications and limitations of conventional anorectal manometry. The second part then focuses on the general concepts of high-resolution manometry and the difference between conventional anorectal manometry and HRAM/HDAM, including technical aspects and different equipment. The third part explains how to perform, analyze, and interpret HRAM and HDAM recordings and describes the parameters study protocol, normal values, and how to formulate a particular diagnosis. Lastly, the fourth part includes a collection of normal and pathological images with a glossary of the most frequently used terms. Written by experts in the field of anorectal manometry and defecation disorders, this book is of interest to specialists and residents dealing with these conditions.

The editor is grateful to all the authors of the different chapters who with passion, intelligence, and patience shared their knowledge and their experience to produce a text that could be useful to all those who want to approach this new technology or improve their own knowledge.

Pisa, Italy   Massimo Bellini

Contents

Anorectal Functional Anatomy

1

Filippo Pucciani

Knowledge of anorectal functional anatomy is the preliminary conceptual acquisition for understanding both the pathophysiology of defecation disorders and the instrumental data provided by anorectal manometry.

In order to give an orderly presentation of the topic and to facilitate the acquisition of anatomical notions, the topic will be divided into functional anatomy of the anal canal, functional anatomy of the rectum and, finally, functional anatomy of the pelvic floor. The anatomical description of bones, nerves, arteries, veins, and lymphatics will be omitted because they are not specifically related to functional evacuative anatomy: they will be described when linked to specific functional activities of visceral structures.

1.1 Functional Anatomy of the Anal Canal

The anal region is separated into the anal canal, the perianal region, and the skin. The anal canal is the terminal segment of the alimentary tract, and lies entirely below the level of the pelvic floor in the region termed the perineum. The anal canal is classically proposed as the anatomical anal canal or the surgical anal canal (Fig. 1.1). The first, the anatomical anal canal, is confined between the anal verge and the dentate line. Its mucous layer is covered by a layered non-keratinized squamous epithelium which presents a smooth appearance. There is profuse innervation with a variety of specialized sensory nerve endings: Meissner's corpuscles which record touch sensation, Krause end-bulbs which respond to thermal stimuli, Golgi-Mazzoni bodies and Pacinian corpuscles which respond to changes in tension and pressure, and genital corpuscles which respond to friction [2]. In addition, there are large diameter free nerve endings sensitive to pain within the epithelium [2]. The

F. Pucciani (✉)
Department of Experimental and Clinical Medicine, University of Florence, Florence, Italy
e-mail: filippo.pucciani@unifi.it

© Springer Nature Switzerland AG 2020
M. Bellini (ed.), *High Resolution and High Definition Anorectal Manometry*,
https://doi.org/10.1007/978-3-030-32419-3_1

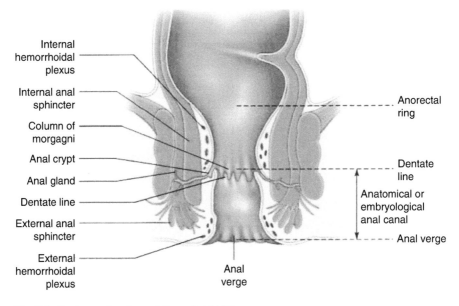

Fig. 1.1 Rectum and anal canal. From Zutshi [1]

anatomical anal canal is about 2.5–3 cm long. The surgical anal canal is longer, about 4–4.5 cm, placed between the anal verge and the apexes of Morgagni rectal columns: it corresponds to the functional length of the high resting pressure zone that is present in the anal canal and it represents the surface entity to be considered for sphincter-saving operations. The epithelium above the dentate line is similar to the glandular epithelial lining of the rectal mucosa and is made up of columnar cells, crypts, and goblet cells. It is relatively insensitive to pain and no specific sensory receptors have been detected through histological examination of the rectum in humans [2, 3].

The submucosal layer of anal canal contains hemorrhoidal tissue that is arranged on the whole circumference (360°) of the anal wall but is also assembled in three cushions respectively in the left lateral position (at 3.00), the right anterior position (at 7.00), and the right posterior position (at 11.00). This spatial arrangement helps to seal the lumen of the anal canal and determines approximately 5–10% of anal resting pressure (ARP). The hemorrhoidal tissue is fixed to the internal anal sphincter by means of fibromuscular fibers (Treitz's muscle): destructive changes in this supporting connective tissue within the anal hemorrhoidal cushions is the paramount condition of hemorrhoidal prolapse.

Where the rectum passes through the pelvic diaphragm, the puborectalis portion of the levator ani muscles fuses with the longitudinal muscle coat of the rectum and, together with the deepest portion of the external sphincter, forms a prominent fibromuscular ring that is called the anorectal ring [4]. The anal canal passes downwards and backwards from its beginning at the anorectal ring, forming almost a right angle (anorectal angle: ARA, approximately 90°) with the termination of the rectum.

The surgical anal canal wall is formed by mucosa, submucosa, and muscular structures including the internal anal sphincter (IAS), the external anal sphincter (EAS), the joined longitudinal muscle, and the puborectalis portion of the levator ani muscle.

1.1.1 Internal Anal Sphincter (IAS)

The IAS is an extension of the inner circular smooth muscle layer of the rectum [3]. It is wrapped superiorly by the puborectalis portion of the levator ani muscle, then more distally by the superficial external sphincter muscle (an extension of the ano-coccygeal ligament), and subsequently by the subcutaneous external striated anal sphincter muscle. Radiologic studies by means of MRI showed that IAS is approximately 3 cm in length and continually closed by tonic contraction [5]. An anatomic study performed by Uz et al. [6] showed that IAS is composed of flat rings of smooth muscle bundles stacked one on top of the other. The average number of ring-like slats observed was 26.33 ± 2.93 (range = 20–30) and each was covered by its own fascia. The smooth muscle fibers and fascia coalesced at three equidistant points around the anal canal to form three columns that extended distally into the lumen. At rest the ring-like slats have a spatially organized structure as horizontal leaves inside the columns and play an important role in closing the lumen of the anal canal, thus assisting anal continence. During defecation the three columns are pulled peripherally toward the fibromuscular band of joined longitudinal muscle, the ring-like slats become vertical, opening the lumen and allowing stool to pass distally. The IAS, as mentioned above, develops important tone for maintaining high anal pressure (70% of ARP) and continence. The mechanism underlying tone generation in the internal anal sphincter is controversial. The hypothesis that tone depends upon generation of electrical slow waves initiated in intramuscular interstitial cells of Cajal (ICC-IM) by activation of Ca^{2+}-activated Cl^- channels and voltage-dependent L-type Ca^{2+} channels has been recently advanced [7]. The inhibition of IAS contractile activity (recto-anal inhibitory reflex: RAIR) would be conversely activated by nitric oxide (NO) release from non-cholinergic non-adrenergic nerve endings. The IAS also has an extrinsic autonomic nerve supply by means of *internal anal sphincter nerves* that emerge from the anterior-inferior edge of the pelvic plexus. They travel within the neurovascular bundle along the inner surface of the levator ani muscle, antero-laterally to the rectum, to penetrate the longitudinal rectal muscle layer just at the fusion line with the pubococcygeal muscle at the anorectal junction to form the conjoint longitudinal muscle. At this point they enter the intersphincteric space to reach the IAS [8]. Their identification and precisely described topographical location provides a basis for nerve-sparing rectal resection procedures and help to prevent postoperative functional anorectal disorders due to internal anal sphincter nerves lesions. Whenever possible, transection of the rectum, during anterior rectal resection with total mesorectum excision, should be done proximal to the conjunction of the pubococcygeal and longitudinal rectal muscle just at the lowermost end of the mesorectum. On the contrary, preservation of these nerves in intersphincteric resections is not usually possible as a rule, because the region of their penetration into the anorectal muscle tube is just a part of the resected specimen [8].

1.1.2 Joined Longitudinal Muscle

The joined longitudinal muscle originates from the fusion of striated muscle fibers of puborectalis muscle with smooth muscle fibers of the longitudinal musculature of the rectum, lying in the intersphincteric space between internal anal sphincter and external anal sphincter and finally ending up melding into fibers that are anchored in the perianal subcutaneous tissue [9]. The muscle's path has suggested that its contraction provokes the corrugation of the anus; for this reason, the muscle is also named "corrugator ani muscle," but its function is very likely to act as an aid during defecation by everting the anus. It is hypothesized also that the joint longitudinal muscle can participate in fecal continence by influencing anal resting pressure but its specific role in this function is unknown.

1.1.3 External Anal Sphincter (EAS)

The EAS is a cylindrical striated muscle under voluntary control and comprises predominantly slow-twitch muscle fibers: it is capable of prolonged contraction but with age there is a shift towards more type II (rapid) fibers [10]. The EAS constitutes the inferior outer aspect of the anal sphincter and envelops the intersphincteric space. The external sphincter is longer and wider than the internal sphincter, and the distal edge of the EAS is normally distal to that of the IAS by at least 1 cm. Between these two edges, it is relatively simple to palpate the intersphincteric groove in the anal verge. Sex-related differences include a significantly shorter external sphincter in women than in men both laterally and anteriorly [11].

The external anal sphincter is conventionally described as consisting of three parts: a subcutaneous part, a superficial part, and a deep part [3] that all act together synergistically. The *subcutaneous* part is included in the perianal subcutaneous tissue, in contact with the external hemorrhoidal plexus and it is crossed by joined longitudinal muscle fibers. The *superficial* part, constituting the main portion of the muscle, arises from a narrow tendinous band, the anococcygeal raphe, which stretches from the tip of the coccyx to the posterior margin of the anus; it forms two flattened planes of muscular tissue, which encircle the anus and meet in front to be inserted into the central tendinous point of the perineum, joining with the superficial transverse perineal muscle, the levator ani, and the bulbocavernosus muscle. The *deep* part is merged with puborectalis muscle behind the rectoanal junction, area that by touch is identified as anorectal ring [12]. The EAS has a resting contraction that contributes about 20% of anal resting pressure. Its functional activity is related to (1) further voluntary muscular recruitment that provides contraction as an emergency continence mechanism, manometrically identified by maximal voluntary contraction (MVC) or to (2) a voluntary relaxation that opens the anal canal during defecation, a function detected by means of the manometric straining test during attempts to strain to defecate [13]. *Shafik* hypothesized that the synergistic activity of the EAS parts may occur by means of a *triple loop system* whereby the muscle spatial organization allows for sealing off or opening the anal canal [14]. EAS activity is controlled by somatic nerves, the right and left inferior rectal nerves, each derived directly from the corresponding pudendal nerve (S2–S4).

1.1.4 Puborectalis Muscle

The puborectalis muscle is the medial part of levator ani muscle, comprised also of pubococcygeus muscle and the iliococcygeus muscle. Muscular fibers of the puborectalis muscle arise from the periosteum on the posterior surface of the pubic bone 1 cm, or more, lateral to the pubic symphysis. These fibers run posteriorly and turn medially behind the rectoanal junction to meet and merge with their counterparts from the other side. Together these fibers form a sling behind the rectoanal junction. The constant tonic contraction in this sling accounts for the sharp rectoanal angle (ARA: $\approx 90°$) but the puborectalis muscle contracts, voluntarily or in response to any sudden increase in intra-abdominal pressure, to prevent incontinence. With contraction, the anorectum is displaced anteriorly and the anorectal angle changes, becoming more acute. On the contrary, voluntary relaxation of the puborectalis sling allows straightening of the rectoanal tube, a mandatory prerequisite to defecation. The puborectalis muscle borders and supports the urogenital hiatus in which the urethra, vagina, and anorectum lie: contraction of the puborectalis leads to narrowing of the urogenital hiatus.

Cadaveric studies showed that the puborectalis muscle is mainly innervated (76.5%) by the pudendal nerve branches [15].

There is a particular anatomical continuity between the deep part of the external anal sphincter and the puborectalis muscle. Their muscular fibers are practically inseparable and one point of discussion is the contribution of the puborectalis muscle to the anal sphincter. MRI studies have clarified that the external sphincter forms the lower outer part of the anal sphincter and the puborectalis the upper outer part [11, 16]. From a functional point of view, it is not clear whether the contraction/relaxation activity of the two muscles is always synchronous or not.

1.2 Functional Anatomy of the Rectum

The rectosigmoid junction is in front of the sacral promontory. The rectum begins at the level of the sacral promontory at a point where the taenia coli fuse to form a continuous longitudinal muscle layer. At this point, the rectum is the direct continuation of the sigmoid colon. It descends along the curve of the sacral hollow to the level of the levator ani and then turns downwards and posteriorly through the anorectal ring where it becomes continuous with the anal canal. In addition to displaying the ventral bend, the rectum possesses a succession of three, smooth, laterally facing curves. The upper and lower curves are directed to the right and the middle curve to the left. Each of the three "curves" possesses, on its luminal aspect, a transverse, sickle-shaped fold known as a rectal shelf or *"Houston valve"*: these three folds are produced by the thickened muscle in the rectal wall covered with overlying mucosa. According to the arrangement of the Houston valves, the rectum can be divided into three parts: the lower third (*low rectum*), about 5 cm long, from the upper edge of the anatomical anal canal to the lower rectal valve, the middle third, 3–4 cm long from lower rectal valve to the medial rectal valve, and the upper third (*high rectum*), about 4 cm long, from the medial rectal valve to the upper rectal valve. The rectum, therefore, is long about 13 cm, from dentate line to upper rectal valve. The entire length of the rectum (except perhaps the very distal centimeter) is surrounded by a cuff of fat termed *perirectal fat*, which is generally more abundant posteriorly than anteriorly. The parietal peritoneum forms the Douglas hollow with the peritoneal fold at 7–8 cm from the anal verge: at the level below, where the extra-peritoneal rectum begins, perirectal fat is in turn surrounded by a distinct circumferential fascial layer called the *fascia propria* of the rectum. The fascia propria enclosing the perirectal fat with the contained lymph nodes is referred to as the *mesorectum*, anatomical structure that must be removed to perform the total mesorectal excision (TME) which involves surgical timing during operations for low rectal cancer.

The rectum has a tonic parietal adaptation to its content for which it is not possible to define its absolute volumetric capacity. Different endoluminal volumes trigger different rectal sensations that may be detected by means of anorectal manometry: the minimal perception of a fecal bolus (CRST: conscious rectal sensitivity threshold), the constant perception with desire to defecate or call to stool (CS: constant sensation), the unbearable distressing defecatory perception (MTV: maximal tolerated volume) [17]. Response of the wall to increasing endoluminal volumes is, on the contrary, evaluated by means of rectal compliance that is expressed by a curve built from the $\Delta V/\Delta P$ results.

1.3   Functional Anatomy of the Pelvic Floor

The term pelvic floor refers to the set of muscles, ligaments, and fascial structures that cover the external opening of the pelvis. Therefore, the pelvic floor is made up of different components placed between the peritoneum and the perineal skin: from top to bottom these are the peritoneum, pelvic viscera, endopelvic fascia, levator ani muscles, perineal membrane, and perineal muscles. The pelvic organs are often thought of as being supported by the pelvic floor, but are actually a part of it. For example, the uterus plays an important role in forming the pelvic floor through their connections to side pelvic walls by means of cardinal and uterosacral ligaments.

Schematically, the pelvic floor can be divided into a deep plane (pelvic diaphragm and urogenital diaphragm) and a superficial plane (perineum).

1.3.1 Levator Ani Muscles

When levator ani muscles (iliococcygeus, pubococcygeus, and puborectalis muscles) and their covering fascia (part of endopelvic fascia) are considered together, the combined structures are defined as the *pelvic diaphragm*. The median opening of the pelvic diaphragm is defined as the levator ani hiatus and is crossed in the anterior/posterior direction by the bladder, uterus, and rectum in woman, and by the bladder and rectum in man. The perineal membrane or *urogenital diaphragm*, a dense triangular membrane of connective tissue that surrounds the urethra, is placed anteriorly, in a lower layer, between the branches of the pelvic diaphragm.

Levator ani muscles are mainly composed of three muscles per side that blend together. The iliococcygeus muscle originates from tendinous arch of the levator ani and the two sides fuse medially in the anococcygeal raphe. The pubococcygeus muscle (also known as the pubo-visceral muscle) attaches the pelvic organs to the pubic bone: it arises from the anterior half of the tendinous arch and the periosteum of the posterior surface of the pubic bone at the lower border of the pubic symphysis and its fibers are directed posteriorly and are inserted into the anococcygeal raphe and coccyx. The puborectalis muscle originates about 1 cm from the pubic symphysis, in a posterior direction; it surrounds the rectum and thus forms a sling behind it. There are also lesser-known levator ani subdivisions that are called pubovaginal, puboanal, and puboperineal muscles. None of these levator ani muscles is delimited with respect to each other but forms a continuous muscular layer with a medial hole, lying down like a diaphragm from one side of the pelvis to the other. It is easy to imagine how the contraction and relaxation of these muscles should be synchronous and coordinated.

By restricting the topic only to the function of the posterior pelvic area, relative to rectum and anus, the levator ani muscles interact all together in the mechanisms of fecal continence and defecation.

Endoanal electromyographic measurements using Multiple Array Probe Leiden (MAPLe) [18] showed that it may be possible to register the electromyographic activity of different muscles of the pelvic floor and their sides, but the data refer only to resting state and anal squeezing: evacuation cannot be detected because the probe is expelled. The function of puborectalis muscle has been described above. Dynamic MRI suggests that, at the evacuative phase of defecation, relaxation of the puborectalis muscle frees the posterior rectal wall while simultaneous contraction of the pubococcygeus muscle pulls the anterior rectal wall forward, further increasing the diameter of the rectum and thereby reducing internal anorectal resistance to the expulsion of feces [19]. Iliococcygeus muscle activity is known only in relation to its contraction: studies with dynamic MRI have shown that the basic tone of the iliococcygeus gives it a dome shape, and that the muscle has a reflex contraction against abdominal strain that ensures the anal continence [20].

1.3.2   Perineum

The perineum is the region containing fat and muscles below the pelvic diaphragm extending to the perineal skin. The perineum has topographically a lozenge shape, delimited bilaterally by a line that goes from the pubic symphysis to the ischial tuberosity and from this to the tip of the coccyx. A transversal line, between ischial tuberosities, divides the perineum into two triangles, an anterior, urogenital one containing urethra and vagina in woman and only the urethra in men, and a posterior, anal triangle.

The perineum has a superficial and a deep layer. The superficial plane (Fig. 1.2), limited by the superficial perineal fascia, contains the perineal body and bilateral superficial muscles, some of which are placed around the genital system (bulbospongiosus, ischiocavernosus, and the *superficial transverse perinei* muscles) and others of which are placed around the anal canal (external anal sphincter). All these muscles, excluding the ischiocavernosus muscle, are anchored medially to the perineal body, a fibrous tissue structure placed halfway between the anal verge and the posterior commissure of the labia majora, on which the rectovaginal septum and the levator ani muscle also converge. The deep perineal plane includes the *deep transverse perinei* and the compressor urethra. Superficial and deep transverse perinei muscles, according to their insertions, have active supporting properties for visceral canals that pass through perineum and participate in the post-defecation reflex. This reflex is the muscular repositioning response after the evacuative slop of the pelvic floor and its impairment is probably the first pathophysiologic element of descending perineum syndrome [21].

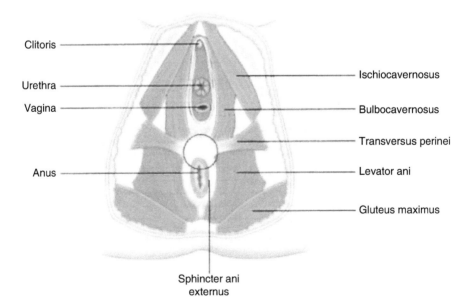

Clitoris

Urethra

Vagina

Anus

Ischiocavernosus

Bulbocavernosus

Transversus perinei

Levator ani

Gluteus maximus

Sphincter ani externus

Fig. 1.2 Perineum: superficial plane. From [1]

In conclusion, the functional anatomy of the structures that participate in bowel movements is complex: the anatomical relationships of these structures explain the functional coordination that underlies fecal continence and defecation. Similarly, knowledge of the spatial arrangement of the viscera and their interaction with the musculofascial structures is crucial for the correct interpretation of lesions relating to the static and dynamics pathologic positions of the viscera.

References

1. Zutshi M, editor. Anorectal disease. Cham: Springer; 2016.
2. Rogers J. Testing for and the role of anal and rectal sensation. Baillieres Clin Gastroenterol. 1992;6:179–91.
3. Mahadevan V. The anatomy of the rectum and anal canal. Surgery. 2010;29:5–10.
4. Morgan CN. The surgical anatomy of the anal canal and rectum. Postgrad Med J. 1936;12:287–300.
5. Kashyap P, Bates N. Magnetic resonance imaging anatomy of the anal canal. Australas Radiol. 2004;48:443–9.
6. Uz A, Elhan A, Ersoy M, Tekdemir I. Internal anal sphincter: an anatomic study. Clin Anat. 2004;7:17–20.
7. Cobine CA, Hannah EE, Zhu MH, Lyle HE, Rock JR, Sanders KM, Ward SM, Keef KD. ANO1 in intramuscular interstitial cells of Cajal plays a key role in the generation of slow waves and tone in the internal anal sphincter. J Physiol. 2017;595:2021–41.
8. Stelzner S, Böttner M, Kupsch J, Kneist W, Quirke P, West NP, Witzigmann H, Wedel T. Internal anal sphincter nerves - a macroanatomical and microscopic description of the extrinsic autonomic nerve supply of the internal anal sphincter. Colorectal Dis. 2018;20:O7–O16.
9. Lunnis S. Anatomy and function of the anal longitudinal muscle. Br J Surg. 1992;79:882–4.
10. Lierse W, Holschneider AM, Steinfeld J. The relative proportions of type I and type II muscle fibres in the external sphincter ani muscle at different ages and stages of development – observations on the development of continence. Eur J Pediatr Surg. 1993;3:28–32.
11. Rociu E, Stoker J, Eijkemans MJ, Laméris JS. Normal anal sphincter anatomy and age- and sex-related variations at high-spatial-resolution endoanal MR imaging. Radiology. 2000;217:395–401.
12. Stoker J. Anorectal and pelvic floor anatomy. Best Pract Res Clin Gastroenterol. 2009;23:463–75.
13. Rao SS, Welcher KD, Leistikow JS. Obstructive defecation: a failure of rectoanal coordination. Am J Gastroenterol. 1998;93:1042–50.
14. Shafik A. A new concept of the anatomy of the anal sphincter mechanism and the physiology of defecation. The external anal sphincter: a triple-loop system. Investig Urol. 1975;12:412–9.
15. Grigorescu BA, Lazarou G, Olson TR, Downie SA, Powers K, Greston WM, Mikhail MS. Innervation of the levator ani muscles: description of the nerve branches to the pubococcygeus, iliococcygeus, and puborectalis muscles. Int Urogynecol J Pelvic Floor Dysfunct. 2008;19:107–16.
16. Hussain SM, Stoker J, Laméris JS. Anal sphincter complex: endoanal MR imaging of normal anatomy. Radiology. 1995;197:671–7.
17. Verkuijl SJ, Trzpis M, · Broens PMA. Normal rectal filling sensations in patients with an enlarged rectum. Dig Dis Sci 2018 64, 1312; doi: https://doi.org/10.1007/s10620-018-5201-6.
18. Voorham-van der Zalm PJ, Voorham JC, van den Bos TW, Ouwerkerk TJ, Putter H, Wasser MN, Webb A, DeRuiter MC, Pelger RC. Reliability and differentiation of pelvic floor muscle

electromyography measurements in healthy volunteers using a new device: the Multiple Array Probe Leiden (MAPLe). Neurourol Urodyn. 2013;3:341–8.

19. Petros P, Swash M, Bush M, Fernandez M, Gunnemann A, Zimmer M. Defecation 1: testing a hypothesis for pelvic striated muscle action to open the anorectum. Tech Coloproctol. 2012;16:437–43.

20. Delmas V, Ami O, Iba-Zizen MT. Dynamic study of the female levator ani muscle using MRI 3D vectorial modeling. Bull Acad Natl Med. 2010;194:969–80.

21. Pucciani F. Descending perineum syndrome: new perspectives. Tech Coloproctol. 2015;19:443–8.

Anorectal Functional Anatomy and Pathophysiology

2

Pathophysiology of Continence and Defecation

Gabrio Bassotti

The control of continence in humans is under voluntary control and, in physiological conditions, each individual is able to determine whether, how, and when to evacuate. Thus, continence and defecation are strictly linked, and their control is probably due to evolutionary and socio-cultural adaptations [1, 2]. Continence mainly depends on anal sphincter function, whereas defecation also involves colonic motility [3]. However, the current understanding of the pathophysiological mechanisms regulating continence and defecation is still incomplete, also due to investigators' disagreement on what is "normality" in such instances.

Defecation is the ultimate result of a concatenation of events that start with the more proximal ileo-colonic motility by means of a sensation of "call to stool" and terminate with the opening of the anal sphincter and the expulsion of stools [4].

Under physiological conditions, there is a close relationship between the forceful colonic propulsive activity, the so-called high-amplitude propagated contractions (HAPC, the manometric equivalent of the radiologically described mass movements) [5], the call to stool, and defecation (Fig. 2.1). However, the exact role of HAPC in the defecatory urge is still debated, and the main role of this forceful activity seems to shift large quantity of endoluminal contents in an oro-aboral direction [6]. This happens through a regional linkage, by means of the overlapping of two consecutive HAPC, that spans the entire large bowel [7]. Together with the cyclical bursts of contractions (periodic colonic motor activity) mainly present in the sigmoid colon [8], the propagated activity modulates the delivery of contents into the rectum. This is facilitated by the fact that distension of the sigmoid causes contraction with concomitant relaxation of the recto-sigmoid junction [9]. Of interest, this relationship between HAPC and the call to stool is often abnormal in chronically constipated patients in whom, compared to controls, a decreased number of HAPC (or their absence) is frequently documented [10, 11].

G. Bassotti (✉)
Gastroenterology and Hepatology Section, Department of Medicine, University of Perugia Medical School, Perugia, Italy

© Springer Nature Switzerland AG 2020
M. Bellini (ed.), *High Resolution and High Definition Anorectal Manometry*,
https://doi.org/10.1007/978-3-030-32419-3_2

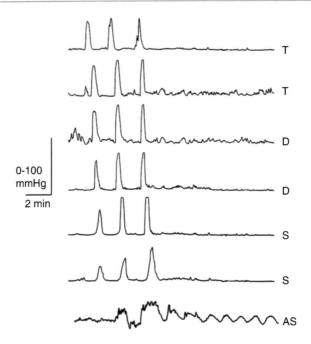

0-100
mmHg

2 min

Fig. 2.1 Representative manometric tracing showing an increase in the number of high-amplitude propagated contractions, spanning the colon and preceding the anal sphincter opening that leads to defecation. Abbreviations: *T* transverse colon, *D* descending colon, *S* sigmoid colon, *AS* anal sphincter

At rest, there is a state of continuous contraction by the external anal sphincter, the puborectalis muscle, and the levator ani; this state helps both to maintain continence and to support the weight of the pelvic viscera [3]. Concerning defecation, the puborectalis muscle probably has the most relevant role, since its traction maintains the anorectal angle at approximately 90°, helping in preservation of the continence. Of interest, its paradoxical contraction during straining is related to one of the main mechanisms of obstructed defecation, the so-called pelvic floor dyssynergia [12].

The first phase of defecation is characterized, as recalled above, by the defecatory urge, and it is preceded by a progressive increase in frequency and amplitude of HAPC [11] (Fig. 2.1). It is currently thought that this sensation is primarily originated in the rectum [3], as demonstrated by the fact that progressive rectal distension causes a graded sensory response that starts with an awareness of filling [13]. Continuing the distension, there is the onset of a constant sensation (often described as the desire to pass flatus) progressively replaced by an urge to defecate when the maximum tolerable volume is reached [14, 15]. However, the urge sensation may also originate extra-rectally, from the stimulation of nerve endings and stretch receptors of the pelvic floor muscles (including the puborectalis muscle) and from structures adjacent to the rectum [16].

The rectum fills during the predefecatory phase. In normal conditions, the rectal ampulla accommodates to increased volumes with a small change in pressure (adaptive relaxation) [17], allowing it to temporarily store the contents until defecation is socially convenient. A reduced perception of the call to stool and constipation are frequently associated with an impaired perception of rectal distension (rectal hyposensitivity) [17]; this can lead to overflow incontinence [14]. On the other hand, an increased perception of distension (i.e., rectal hypersensitivity) is found in patients with urgency, with or without fecal incontinence [18]. An appropriate response to the call to stool, needing intact neurophysiological and biomechanical activity, is of a paramount importance for a correct evacuation, and it may be attenuated by the habitual suppression of the defecatory stimulus. This may ultimately result in fecal impaction up to the development of a secondary megarectum when the stimulus suppression is repeated in the time course [19].

It is still uncertain whether the anal canal contributes to the generation of the defecatory urge, since the distension of a balloon in the anal canal elicits a sensation of "stool escape" from the anus rather than an urge to defecate [20]. The anal canal chiefly provides a tight seal throughout the day, except when the subject decides to pass winds or wants to defecate; the major contribution to this sealing is due to the internal anal sphincter (IAS) [3, 21], and its intact sensation is essential for the sampling reflex [22].

The sampling reflex and the defecatory urge, in turn, are then determinants of the expulsive phase and, if the subject decides that it is socially or otherwise appropriate, a variable amount of rectal and colonic contents are expelled with the additional help of voluntary straining and adoption of an appropriate defecatory posture [3]. Thus, once defecation is decided, stool expulsion happens by means of increased endorectal pressure, relaxation of the pelvic floor, and relaxation of the anal canal. Concerning the role of endorectal pressure, the available data are not univocal, and it is likely that stool expulsion also needs help from more proximal colorectal contractions, depending on the volume and consistence of the stools [23]. More data are available on the important role of an adequate pelvic floor and anal canal relaxation as main mechanisms for effective expulsion of feces. In fact, the coupling of pelvic floor relaxation with increased intra-abdominal pressures causes the lowering of the pelvic floor, which assumes a funnel shape with its tip at the anorectal junction. The anorectal angle therefore straightens following the relaxation of the puborectalis and the posture (often squatting or semi-squatting) assumed during defecation; the concomitant relaxation of the anal canal allows the fecal matter to be expelled (Fig. 2.2). The involuntary relaxation of the internal anal sphincter follows the distention of the rectum; of interest, this relaxation is also proportional to the intrarectal pressure [21] (Fig. 2.3). The pathophysiological importance of these mechanisms is demonstrated by the fact that inadequate pelvic floor and anal canal relaxation are well recognized causes of disordered defecation (pelvic floor dyssynergia, dyssynergic defecation subtype) [24].

Termination of defecation starts semi-voluntarily with the sense of complete rectal emptying, followed by the contraction of the external anal sphincter and the pelvic floor; their contraction allows the closure of the anal canal and re-directs the pressure gradient towards the rectum [3]. Finally, the "closing reflex" (a transient pressure increase following the passage of stools) of the external sphincter provides

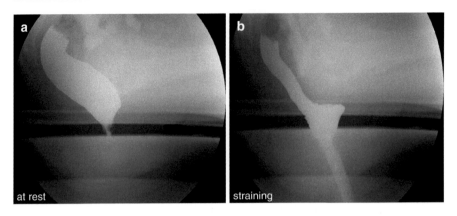

Fig. 2.2 Representative defecographic images showing rectal dynamics at rest (**a**) and under straining (**b**). Note that in (**b**) the individual straightens the anorectal angle allowing most of the rectal content to be expelled

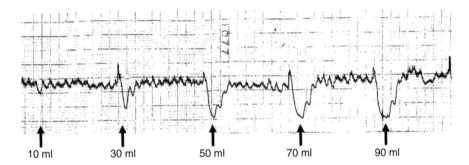

10 ml   30 ml   50 ml   70 ml   90 ml

Fig. 2.3 Representative manometric tracing showing relaxation of the anal sphincter following progressive rectal balloon distention. Note that the amount of relaxation is proportional to the volume of rectal distention

time to the internal sphincter to recover its tone [25]. After the individual terminates to strain, intra-abdominal pressure decreases and the postural reflex of the pelvic floor is reactivated [26], with the increased traction of the puborectalis muscle on the anorectal junction that causes to re-establish the basal state of the angle. The concomitant elongation of the anal canal also causes the passive distention of the anal cushions, thus resulting in the complete closure of the anal canal [3].

The knowledge, although incomplete, of the pathophysiological mechanisms underlying continence and defecation has practical implications, and has led to the classification of anorectal disorders according to the Rome criteria, now present in literature in their fourth version [27] (Table 2.1). In fact, the pathophysiological grounds of these disorders may basically be reconducted to the dysfunction, single or in association, of the anal sphincter (abnormal pressure or relaxation), of the pelvic floor (abnormal dynamics), and of the rectum (abnormal contraction or perception).

Table 2.1 Rome IV classification of anorectal disorders (adapted from reference [27])

Functional anorectal disorders
– Fecal incontinence
– Functional anorectal pain (including levator ani syndrome, unspecified functional anorectal pain, and proctalgia fugax)
– Functional defecation disorders (including dyssynergic defecation and inadequate defecatory propulsion)

References

1. Bassotti G, Villanacci V. The control of defecation in humans: an evolutionary advantage? Tech Coloproctol. 2013;17:623–4. https://doi.org/10.1007/s10151-013-1037-4.
2. Bassotti G, Müller-Lissner S. Controlling defecation: to be (predator) or not to be (prey), that is the question.... Z Gastroenterol. 2015;53:460–2. https://doi.org/10.105 5/s-0034-1399242.
3. Palit S, Lunniss PJ, Scott SM. The physiology of human defecation. Dig Dis Sci. 2012;57:1445–64. https://doi.org/10.1007/s10620-012-2071-1.
4. Bassotti G, de Roberto G, Castellani D, Sediari L, Morelli A. Normal aspects of colorectal motility and abnormalities in slow transit constipation. World J Gastroenterol. 2005;11:2691–6.
5. Narducci F, Bassotti G, Gaburri M, Morelli A. Twenty four hour manometric recording of colonic motor activity in healthy man. Gut. 1987;28:17–25.
6. Bassotti G, Iantorno G, Fiorella S, Bustos-Fernandez L, Bilder CR. Colonic motility in man: features in normal subjects and in patients with chronic idiopathic constipation. Am J Gastroenterol. 1999;94:1760–70.
7. Dinning PG, Zarate N, Szczesniak MM, Mohammed SD, Preston SL, Fairclough PD, Lunniss PJ, Cook IJ, Scott SM. Bowel preparation affects the amplitude and spatiotemporal organization of colonic propagating sequences. Neurogastroenterol Motil. 2010;22:633–e176. https://doi.org/10.1111/j.1365-2982.2010.01480.x.
8. Rao SS, Sadeghi P, Beaty J, Kavlock R, Ackerson K. Ambulatory 24-h colonic manometry in healthy humans. Am J Physiol Gastrointest Liver Physiol. 2001;280:G629–39.
9. Shafik A. Sigmoido-rectal junction reflex: role in the defecation mechanism. Clin Anat. 1996;9:391–4.
10. Bassotti G, Gaburri M, Imbimbo BP, Rossi L, Farroni F, Pelli MA, Morelli A. Colonic mass movements in idiopathic chronic constipation. Gut. 1988;29:1173–9.
11. Dinning PG, Bampton PA, Andre J, Kennedy ML, Lubowski DZ, King DW, Cook IJ. Abnormal predefecatory colonic motor patterns define constipation in obstructed defecation. Gastroenterology. 2004;127:49–56.
12. Bassotti G, Chistolini F, Sietchiping-Nzepa F, de Roberto G, Morelli A, Chiarioni G. Biofeedback for pelvic floor dysfunction in constipation. BMJ. 2004;328:393–6.
13. Meunier P, Mollard P, Marechal JM. Physiopathology of megarectum: the association of megarectum with encopresis. Gut. 1976;17:224–7.
14. Sun WM, Read NW, Miner PB. Relation between rectal sensation and anal function in normal subjects and patients with faecal incontinence. Gut. 1990;31:1056–61.
15. Broens PM, Penninckx FM, Lestár B, Kerremans RP. The trigger for rectal filling sensation. Int J Color Dis. 1994;9:1–4.
16. Scharli AF, Kiesewetter WB. Defecation and continence: some new concepts. Dis Colon Rectum. 1970;13:81–107.
17. Gladman MA, Aziz Q, Scott SM, Williams NS, Lunniss PJ. Rectal hyposensitivity: pathophysiological mechanisms. Neurogastroenterol Motil. 2009;21:508–16. https://doi.org/10.1111/j.1365-2982.2008.01216.x.

18. Chan CL, Scott SM, Williams NS, Lunniss PJ. Rectal hypersensitivity worsens stool frequency, urgency, and lifestyle in patients with urge fecal incontinence. Dis Colon Rectum. 2005;48:134–40.
19. Mimura T, Nicholls T, Storrie JB, Kamm MA. Treatment of constipation in adults associated with idiopathic megarectum by behavioural retraining including biofeedback. Color Dis. 2002;4:477–82.
20. Goligher JC, Hughes ES. Sensibility of the rectum and colon. Its rôle in the mechanism of anal continence. Lancet. 1951;1:543–7.
21. Frenckner B. Function of the anal sphincters in spinal man. Gut. 1975;16:638–44.
22. Miller R, Lewis GT, Bartolo DC, Cervero F, Mortensen NJ. Sensory discrimination and dynamic activity in the anorectum: evidence using a new ambulatory technique. Br J Surg. 1988;75:1003–7.
23. Bharucha AE. Pelvic floor: anatomy and function. Neurogastroenterol Motil. 2006;18:507–19.
24. Bharucha AE, Wald A, Enck P, Rao S. Functional anorectal disorders. Gastroenterology. 2006;130:1510–8.
25. Nyam DC. The current understanding of continence and defecation. Singap Med J. 1998;39:132–6.
26. Porter NH. A physiological study of the pelvic floor in rectal prolapse. Ann R Coll Surg Engl. 1962;31:379–404.
27. Rao SC, Bharucha AE, Chiarioni G, Felt-Bersma R, Knowles C, Malcolm A, Wald A. Anorectal disorders. Gastroenterology. 2016;150:1430–42. https://doi.org/10.1053/j.gastro.2016.02.009.

Paola Iovino, Maria Cristina Neri, Antonella Santonicola,
and Giuseppe Chiarioni

3.1 Introduction

Anorectal physiology is very complex ensuring evacuation of bowel contents that is highly regulated and requires coordinated function of the colon, rectum, and anus [1].

Dysfunction of anorectum can lead to fecal incontinence that implies the inability to completely control defecation and/or symptoms of an evacuation disorder. Both of them can have a devastating effect on quality of life, involving in North America about 12–19% of the population [2–4].

The underlying etiology and pathophysiology of fecal incontinence and evacuation disorders are multifactorial. Although there are data demonstrating a pivotal role of clinical examination alone to treat these patients [5, 6], with the recent advances in diagnostic technologies, a symptom-based assessment seems unsatisfactory to direct therapy [7–9].

COI: Consulting/Speaker Board: Alfa-Sigma, Allergan, Kiowa-Kirin, Malesci, Omeopiacenza, Takeda and Membership: Anorectal Committee of the Rome Foundation, International Anorectal Physiology Working Group, Conservative Management Committee for Faecal Incontinence of the International Consultation on Incontinence.

P. Iovino (✉) · A. Santonicola
Gastrointestinal Unit, Department of Medicine, Surgery and Dentistry, University of Salerno, Salerno, Italy
e-mail: piovino@unisa.it

M. C. Neri
Division of Gastroenterology and Endoscopy, Geriatric Institute Pio Albergo Trivulzio, Milan, Italy

G. Chiarioni
Division of Gastroenterology B, AOUI Verona, Verona, Italy

Division of Gastroenterology and Hepatology and UNC Center for Functional GI and Motility Disorders, University of North Carolina at Chapel Hill, Chapel Hill, NC, USA

© Springer Nature Switzerland AG 2020
M. Bellini (ed.), *High Resolution and High Definition Anorectal Manometry*,
https://doi.org/10.1007/978-3-030-32419-3_3

As a consequence, the importance of anorectal physiologic testing is increasing more and more [10, 11]. Moreover, there are some studies which outlined that testing anorectal function influences clinical decision and even more, these tests are able to act as biomarkers predicting the response to treatment [12–15].

Ideally, all understood and measurable components that contribute toward continence or defecation should be assessed (Table 3.1). Nevertheless, no single test is able to fully characterize all components that cause fecal incontinence and/or evacuation disorders. This causes controversies on the usefulness of single test; however, when anorectal function assessment is available its clinical utility increases if it is performed in a structured and systematic manner [16].

Table 3.1 Clinical utility of diagnostic tests of anorectal physiological function [3]

Function	Investigation	Clinical use (utility)
Anus		
Motor	Anorectal manometry (conventional)	++++
	Anorectal manometry (high resolution)	++++
	Anorectal manometry (3D)	+++
	Electromyography	+++
	Pudendal nerve terminal motor latency	+
Structure	Endoanal ultrasonography	++++
	Transperineal ultrasonography	+++
	Endoanal or pelvic MRI	+++
	MRI muscle fiber tracking	+
	Electrostimulation	+
Sensory	Light-touch stimulation	+
	Anal evoked potentials	++
Rectum		
Sensory	Balloon distention	++++
	Rectal barostat	+++
	Rectal motor evoked potentials	++
Motor	Distal colonic manometry	++
	Rectal barostat	+++
	Rectal motor evoked potentials	+
Anorectal unit		
Motor, sensory	Anorectal manometry (conventional, high resolution, or 3D)	++++
	Balloon expulsion	++++
Motor, sensory, and structure	Barium defecography	++++
	Magnetic resonance defecography	+++
	Functional lumen imaging probe	+

+ Limited clinical utility or of research interest only
++ Emerging technology with limited data of clinical utility
+++ Recognized clinical utility but less commonly performer
++++ Good clinical utility and commonly performer

Anorectal manometry is the most established and widely available investigative tool, because it is able to detect functional diseases of anal sphincter and/or recto-anal coordination [17–19].

However, it is not a first level diagnostic technique, but it must be used after other morphological methods (radiological and/or endoscopic) had already excluded lesions of the large intestine and in particular rectum-anus. In clinical practice, in subjects with evacuation disorders (fecal incontinence or constipation with difficult evacuation) with no alarm signs (red flags) and symptoms refractory to first-line therapies such as lifestyle modification and optimization of stool consistency, it is justifiable to proceed with anorectal testing [20].

Therefore, in this chapter, the role of anorectal manometry is examined in relation to factors having effects on anorectal pathophysiology.

3.2   Definition

Anorectal manometry is an instrumental investigation able to evaluate the pressure of the anal canal and the distal rectum, providing motor and sensory information on functional phases of defecation and continence of the anorectal tract and of the pelvic floor muscles [17, 18].

It measures the luminal pressure at 6–8 cm above the anal verge and, in particular, it allows to evaluate:

- the high pressure zone (which refers to the length of the anal sphincter muscles);
- the involuntary function of the anal canal at rest,
- the voluntary anal function on squeezing,
- the rectoanal reflexes,
- the rectal sensitivity and compliance,
- the rectoanal coordination during simulated defecation ("push"),
- the capacity to expel a balloon [21–24].

3.3   Equipment for Conventional Manometry

Conventional anorectal manometry is a water perfusion system able to detect pressure values and stimulators of visceral sensitivity receptors existing in the rectal ampoule and in the anal canal.

It consists of four components: a probe, a pressure recording device (amplifier/recorder, pneumohydraulic pump, pressure transducers), a device for displaying the recording (monitor, printer, or chart recorder), and a data storage facility (computer, chart recorder) (Fig. 3.1) [17].

The manometric probes are represented by catheters with internal channels and perfused lateral openings with continuous flow of bi-distilled water or balloon catheters perfused with water or air (Fig. 3.2).

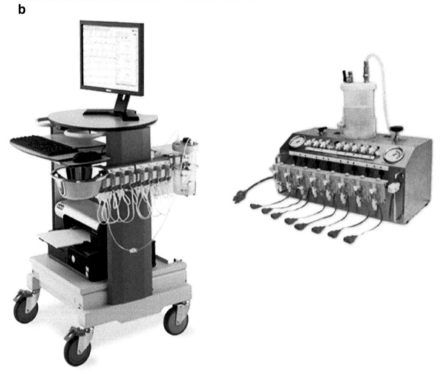

a

A nitrogen tank   C capillary tubing   E manometric catheter
B pressure chamber   D pressure transducer   F amplifier and recorder

b

Fig. 3.1 (**a**) Schematic manometric assembly A nitrogen tank   B pressure chamber   C capillary tubing D pressure transducer   E manometric catheter   F amplifier and recorder. (**b**) Conventional anorectal manometric equipment

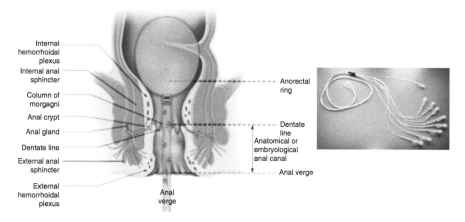

Fig. 3.2 Probe for conventional anorectal manometry

Anorectal manometry can be performed using different types of probes and pressure recording devices. Satisfactory measurements can be obtained also with solid-state microtransducers [25].

3.4 Anorectal Manometry Technique

The patient (who should not be fasting, but must do an evacuation enema a few hours before the examination) is placed in left lateral decubitus with overlapping thighs and bent at 90° on the trunk; the catheter is introduced into the rectum after calibration at the level of the anus.

A run-in period (about 5 min) should be performed to allow the patient relaxing and sphincter tone returning to its physiologic baseline [26].

The integrity of anal sphincter function is assessed by measurement of resting sphincter pressure, the functional length of the anal canal, and squeeze sphincter pressure.

1. Anal resting tone and the functional length of anal canal

    During the first phase of anorectal manometry, the extraction of the probe manually in 1 cm steps (stationary pull-through technique) or at constant speed using an automatic extractor arm (motor pull-through technique) allows to evaluate the functional length of the anal canal and the anal resting tone.

    The functional length of anal canal (high pressure zone, HPZ) is defined as a region (or length) over which resting pressures are ≥30% higher than rectal pressure [27].

We can calculate the mean resting anal pressure since it is the average of all the pressures detected in the HPZ and, the maximal resting anal pressure, defined as the difference between intrarectal pressure and the highest recorded anal sphincter pressure at rest, generally recorded 1–2 cm from the anal verge. Physiologically the anal resting tone is predominantly due to internal anal sphincter (IAS) activity (55–80%, most due to nerve-activity and the remainder purely myogenic) [28], expression of an involuntary function, and to a lesser extent external anal sphincter (30%) and hemorrhoidal pads (15%). Resting sphincter pressure varies according to age, sex, and techniques used. Usually, pressures are higher in men and younger subjects, but with considerable overlap [18, 29, 30].

According to perfused catheter anorectal manometry, the recorded anal canal is often asymmetric. In the proximal anal canal, anterior quadrant pressures are lower than the other quadrants at rest while distally, posterior quadrant pressures are reduced, and in the mid anal canal radial pressures are generally equal in all quadrants [26, 29, 31]. Furthermore, conventional anorectal manometry allows to obtain, through a specific software, the two-dimensional reconstruction of the pressure profile of the anal canal (vector volume) with a detailed evaluation of the pressure asymmetries caused by possible sphincter anatomic pathologies. However, these data are today better obtained through three-dimensional sphincter ultrasound [32].

2. Maximal squeeze pressure and maximal squeeze duration

    During the second phase of anorectal manometry patients were asked to squeeze the anus as hard as possible, avoiding contracting the accessory muscles and, in particular, limiting gluteal muscle involvement. Moreover, the squeeze should be maintained for 30 s, to obtain a measure of fatigability of the external anal sphincter (EAS) [17]; during the squeeze maneuver, the maximal voluntary pressure is recorded at each station to detect appropriate external sphincter activity.

    The maximal squeeze pressure is measured by evaluating the difference between the pressure increments during a maximal voluntary contraction and the basal resting tone at the same level of the anal canal [8, 17, 27].

    The sphincter endurance is the time interval at which the patient is able to maintain a squeeze pressure above the resting pressure, in particular greater than or equal to 50% of the maximum squeeze recorded pressure [17, 27, 33].

    Both of these measurements primarily reflect the strength and fatigability of the EAS [11, 19, 33, 34].

3. The integrity of neural reflex pathway is assessed by measurement of anocutaneous reflex, cough reflex, and rectoanal inhibitory reflex (RAIR)

    (a) Anocutaneous reflex and cough reflex

        The anocutaneous reflex is detected by crawling a needle on the perianal skin; Valsalva reflex evaluation is obtained by inviting the patient to cough. Specifically, cough increases abdominal pressure and, rectal pressure trigger a reflex contraction of the external anal sphincter. The integrity of Valsava reflex acts to maintain anal continence in urgency. This contraction is recorded with an increase in the pressure obtained by the manometer, and cough pressure is calculated as the difference between the maximum pressure recorded during cough and the resting pressure at the same level in the anal canal. Physiologically, it must be higher than the anal canal.

(b) Rectoanal inhibitory reflex (RAIR)

Rectoanal inhibitory reflex (RAIR) is measured by recording the resting anal pressures during rapid and intermittent inflation of a distal rectal balloon, positioned at the apex of the manometric catheter: the balloon is inflating with air, (10 or 20 mL aliquots, up to about 50–60 cc or higher volumes in some cases with chronic constipation and megarectum); in this way is recorded the threshold volume needed to elicit the reflex.

The rapid distention of the rectum leads to a transient increase in rectal pressure (due to secondary rectal contraction—the rectoanal contractile reflex), followed by a transient increase in anal pressure (due to EAS contraction) and finally a prolonged reduction in anal pressure, due to relaxation of IAS (the rectoanal inhibitory reflex); this last is thought to allow sampling rectal contents by sensory area present in the anal canal, allowing discrimination between flatus and fecal matter (solid, liquid, and gas); conversely, the rectoanal contractile reflex is a compensatory mechanism that allows the maintenance of a positive anal pressure during increase of intraabdominal or intrarectal pressure (e.g., coughing) which is essential for continence [8, 34].

4. The assessment of rectal sensibility and rectal compliance

Testing rectal sensitivity is generally performed with a balloon distention, positioned in the rectum, filled (manually using a hand-held syringe or pump-assisted) with air or water. It is able to record intraballoon pressure expression of rectal pressure and distending volumes by means of incorporating water-perfused catheters or microtransducers. During the test, patient is instructed to report the first sensation that is the minimum rectal volume perceived by the patient, desire to defecate, urgency that is the volume associated with the initial urge to defecate, maximum tolerated volume that is the volume at which the patient experiences discomfort and an intense desire to defecate, and pain. These sensory thresholds are recorded (through the distending volume or less frequently the pressure) [3, 8, 35].

This assessment allows also to calculate rectal compliance from the derived pressure–volume curve: it is defined as the "volume response to an imposed pressure," and represents the change in rectal pressure in response to changes in rectal volume (change in volume divided by change in pressure = $\Delta V/\Delta P$). In response to distention, the rectal wall is able to have an "adaptive relaxation" at the beginning due to its viscoelastic properties and this allows accommodation of significant increases in volume despite low intraluminal pressures, so that continence is guaranteed; continuing distention the rectum becomes more resistant to stretch until the elastic limit is reached and regular contractions start, causing an increase of intrarectal pressure [36, 37].

Despite large variation, in literature there is a high degree of reproducibility about recording sensory thresholds [38, 39], and many consensus statements and technical reviews have attested that this test is useful in the assessment of functional intestinal disorders [16, 18, 34].

Another test to get rectal sensitivity makes use of an electronic barostat. Briefly, the barostat maintains a constant pressure on the inside of a bag containing air by means of feedback. The feedback mechanism consists of a strain gauge connected to an injection/aspiration system by means of a relay. Both the strain gauge and the injection/aspiration system are independently connected by a double-lumen polyvinyl tube, one lumen is used for inflation, the other for monitoring pressure, to a non-elastic, oversized, polyethylene ultrathin bag and so very compliant to avoid any influence on internal pressure. A dial allows the selection of the desired pressure level. Pressure and volume within the bag are continuously recorded [40–42]. Measurement of rectal compliance and capacity using the barostat are more specific than those using balloon, considering that this last needs correction because of its intrinsic elasticity. Although barostat is less available, it is advisable to consider it in patients with alterations of rectal sensation already assessed by balloon distention and/or with a strong suspicion of abnormal rectal compliance or capacity [17, 33].

5. The assessment of attempted defecation.

In patients with symptoms of disordered evacuation, the manometric assessment of rectoanal coordination during defecatory maneuvers can help in the diagnosis.

During this part of anorectal testing, the patient is asked to strain or bear down, as during defecation, while pressures of anus and rectum are detected simultaneously; normally an increase in intrarectal pressure is detected, due to the Valsava maneuver, associated with a decrease in intraanal pressure, due to coordinated relaxation of the EAS; these mechanisms facilitate the process of defecation, allowing propulsive forces to drive stool easier through the anal canal with learned response under voluntary control [20, 21].

When defecation is impaired during ARM is possible to observe inadequate rectal propulsive force and/or inadequate relaxation or paradoxical anal contraction [20, 43–45].

Specifically, four patterns of pressure changes seen in the rectum and anus during attempting defecation have been described [33, 44, 46].

Type 1: increase of rectal propulsive pressure (rise in intraabdominal pressure with generation of an adequate pushing force) with paradoxical increase of anal pressure as well.

Type 2: inadequate rectal propulsive pressure (no increase in intrarectal pressure) with paradoxical anal contraction.

Type 3: adequate rectal propulsive pressure (increase in intrarectal pressure) with absent or incomplete anal relaxation ($\leq20\%$) (i.e., no decrease in anal sphincter pressure).

Type 4: inadequate rectal propulsive pressure and absent or incomplete anal sphincter relaxation ($\leq20\%$) (Fig. 3.3) [44, 46].

Unfortunately, some of that abnormal manometric patterns (for example an abnormal reduced rectoanal pressure gradient) during simulated evacuation are found in more than 50% of the asymptomatic subjects and, therefore, the diagnosis of functional defecation disorders cannot rely only on anorectal manometry [2, 8, 33, 44].

According to Rome III criteria, diagnosis of functional defecation disorders is possible in presence of (1) constipation symptoms, (2) the presence of inadequate rectal propulsive force and/or inadequate relaxation or paradoxical anal contraction at ARM (or electromyography), and (3) at least another positive test among balloon expulsion test or impaired rectal evacuation by imaging [47].

The new Rome IV diagnostic criteria for functional defecation disorders (Table 3.2) incorporates also IBS with constipation patients [48]. In addition, the diagnosis of dyssynergic defecation has been limited to the finding of paradoxical anal contraction at either ARM or pelvic floor electromyography.

3.4.1 Balloon Expulsion Test (BET)

This is the simplest procedure for evaluating a patient's ability to evacuate a stool surrogate. It can be performed alone or to implement ARM results. A 16 F Foley that acts as water-filled balloon is placed in the rectum and filled up with 50 mL of warm water to simulate stool; it is possible to use air in place of water; however, the last is better for a more accurate simulation of a fecal bolus. The patient is invited to push for the expulsion of the device on a commode chair or in a private toilet. Recording the time needed to evacuate the balloon is critical to define normal values.

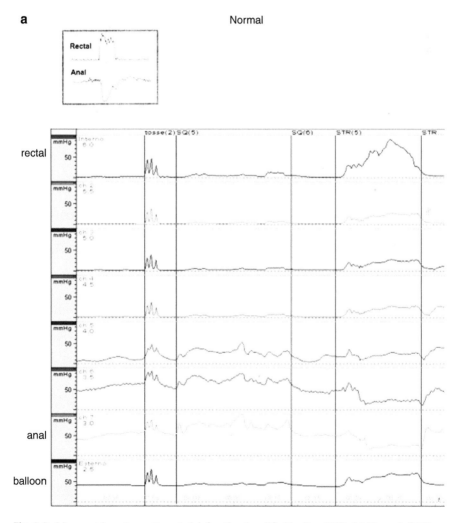

Fig. 3.3 Manometric pattern: attempted defecation (modified by Rao [46]). (**a**) Normal. (**b**) Type I. (**c**) Type II. (**d**) Type III. (**e**) Type IV

b Type I

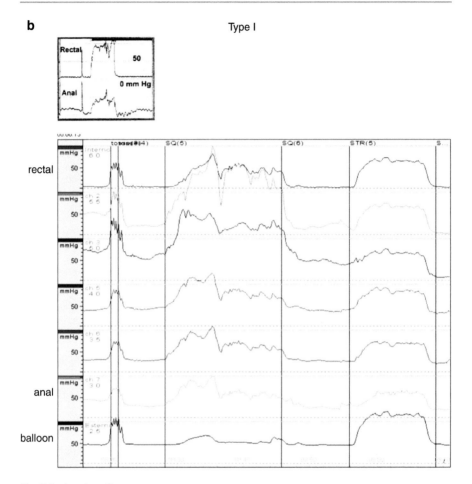

Fig. 3.3 (continued)

c

Type II

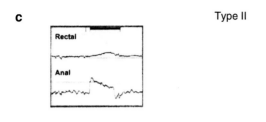

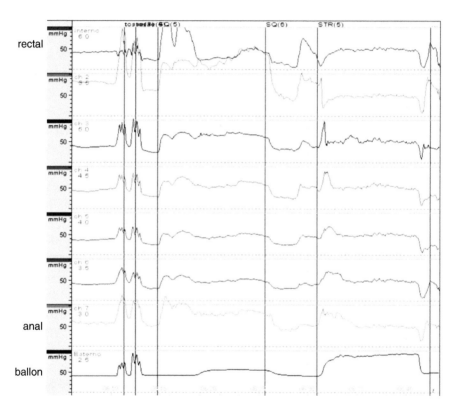

Fig. 3.3 (continued)

d   Type III

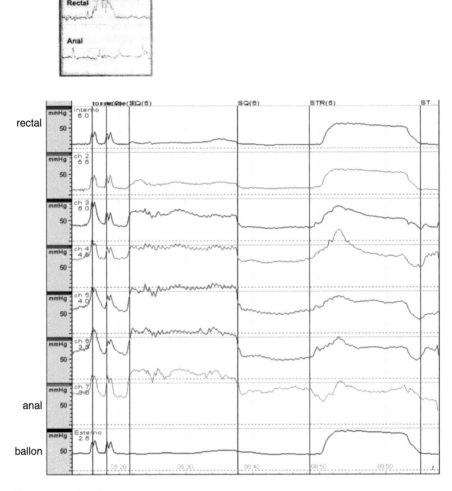

Fig. 3.3 (continued)

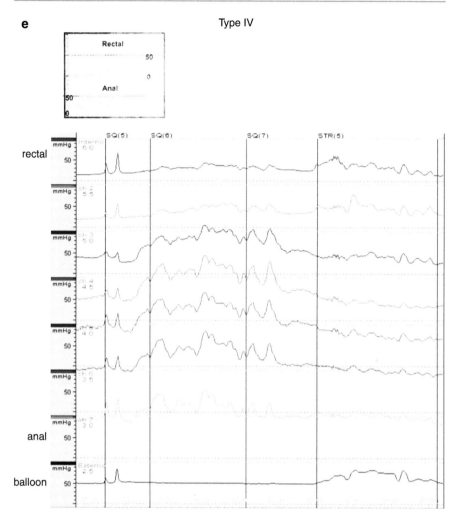

Fig. 3.3 (continued)

Most normal subjects can expel a stool surrogate device within 1 min [8, 20, 49], but although reported cut-off for normality is variable, the generally accepted limit for expulsion is between 1 and 2 min; expulsion times longer than this can suggest defecation disorders or dyssynergic defecation (DD) [8, 33, 49, 50].

ARM should be performed in conjunction with a BET. A recent large cohort study found BET to have a high level of agreement with both ARM and pelvic floor surface electromyography in CC [51].

BET might be performed using the same manometric catheter, at the end of ARM.

Table 3.2 Diagnostic criteria for functional defecation disorders according to Rome IV criteria (modified from [48])

1. The patient must satisfy the diagnostic criteria for functional constipation and or/irritable bowel syndrome-predominant constipation.
2. During repeated attempts to defecate, there must be reduced evacuation characteristics coming from two of the following three tests:
• Anomalous balloon ejection test
• Anomalous model of anorectal evacuation with manometry or EMG of anal surface
• Impairment of evacuation through image acquisition
Criteria should be satisfied for the last 3 months with onset of symptoms at least 6 months before diagnosis
Sub-categories F3a and F3b apply to patients who satisfy the FDD criteria
F3a diagnostic criteria for inadequate defecatory propulsion
Anomalous energy of contraction evaluated with manometry with or without insufficient contraction of the anal sphincter and / or pelvic floor muscles
F3b diagnostic criteria for dyssynergic defecation
Inadequate contraction of the pelvic floor evaluated with EMG of anal surface or manometry with adequate propulsive forces during the defecation
These criteria are described in relation to normal values for the technique appropriate for age and sex

3.4.2 ARM and Pathophysiology

The role of manometric examination allows to recognize multiple mechanisms underlying the most frequent anorectal disease (Table 3.3).

In this part of the chapter, we revise several anorectal disorders enhancing the multiple pathophysiological mechanisms that can be assessed by ARM.

1. Fecal Incontinence (FI)

   FI or involuntary rectal outflow represents the instability to control discharge of gas and stools, with involuntary discharge of them, and occurs when multiple mechanisms of continence (from visceral sensitivity to sphincter tone, to the contractile capacity of striated muscles) are compromised at the same time, even in various ways, so patient reports symptoms like increased frequency or extreme urgency of evacuation, tenesmus, difficulty in holding the stool in case of urgency [56–58].

   The manometric examination is very important in these patients:
   - sphincter hypotonia (low anal resting pressure) that is associated with passive fecal incontinence, often due to degeneration or rupture of smooth muscle ring (IAS activity is the primary component contributing to anal resting tone) [52, 59]. However, ARM may detect very low basal pressures also in continent patients, and in other way incontinent patients may present normal resting tone [22, 60]. As a consequence, measurement of resting tone must be considered in combination with other functional tests [34].
   - symptoms of urge or stress fecal incontinence (urgent need to defecate with inability to arrive to the toilet in time) are often associated with low anal squeeze pressures and suggest strength and fatigue of EAS due to a sphincter

Table 3.3 Pathophysiological mechanism causing fecal incontinence

Function	Investigation	Finding	Examples of disorders
Anus			
Motor	Anorectal manometry	Anal hypotonia	Passive fecal incontinence due to muscular damage (IAS weakness for smooth muscle ring rupture or degeneration): • Obstetric injury • Cauda equina • Myelomeningoceles • Multiple sclerosis • Pudendal neuropathies • Demyelination injury • Diabetes • Spinal cord injury • Stroke • Aging • Dementia/disability • Psychosis • Drugs (laxatives, antidepressants, anticholinergics, caffeine, muscle relaxants) [8, 18, 19]
		Anal hypertonia	Fissures or hemorrhoidal plexuses Chronic constipation [3]
		Anal hypocontractility	Urge or stress fecal incontinence due to EAS weakness for muscular damage: • Obstetric injury (major causative factor) • Neuropathy • Diabetes • Spinal cord injury • Stroke [8, 18, 19, 52]
Rectum			
Sensory	Balloon distension	Rectal hypersensitivity	Urge fecal incontinence Inflammatory bowel diseases Actinic proctitis Rectal neoformation Surgery of the rectum IBS-D [39, 42, 53, 54]
		Rectal hyposensitivity	Fecal impaction (fecal seepage) Chronic constipation Defecation disorders IBS-C Spinal cord injury [8, 35, 50]
Motor sensory and structure	Rectal balloon or barostat	Rectal hypercompliance	Megarectum (lax-floppy rectum) Chronic constipation [50]
		Rectal hypocompliance	Rectal fibrosis (stiff rectum) for chronic ischemia, inflammatory bowel disease (IBD), or pelvic irradiation IBS-D Urge fecal incontinence [8, 34]
Anorectal unit			
Motor	Balloon expulsion	Prolonged expulsion time	Fecal incontinence Chronic constipation
	Anorectal manometry	Anorectal areflexia	Fecal incontinence Hirschsprung's disease Chronic constipation [8, 52, 55]

Irritable bowel disease predominant diarrhea (IBS-D), Irritable bowel syndrome-predominant constipation (IBS-C)

damage (with the major causative factor being obstetric injury) or associated neuropathy [22, 52, 58]. Moreover, also squeeze duration (endurance) is significantly reduced in incontinent patients versus controls [61]; among all measurements of anorectal function, anal squeeze has been shown to have the greatest sensitivity and specificity for discriminating patients with fecal incontinence from continent subjects [8, 60, 62].

- a difference in rectoanal inhibitory reflex compared with controls: the amplitude and duration of this intramural reflex correlate with distending volumes and in clinical practice an abnormal reflex may correlate with clinical or subclinical neuropathy. In particular, in patients with urge incontinence is possible to record an abnormal reflex response, associated with attenuated voluntary squeeze pressure, which could indicate a neural damage of the sacral arc (spinal sacral segments or pudendal nerves); these patients may have a lesion of the cauda equina or sacral plexus, a pudendal neuropathy or a peripheral neuropathy (e.g., diabetes) [19, 34, 63].
- rectal hypersensitivity that can be frequently found in certain patients with urge fecal incontinence [8], as well as in patients with diarrhea-predominant bowel disease (IBS) (the more severe the IBS, the more hypersensitive the patient is) [39, 42, 53, 64]. Rectal hypersensitivity can also be associated with a reduction in the distensibility of the rectum ("stiff" rectum), with symptoms like urgency and frequent defecation, for example in rectum with fibrosis (i.e., inflammatory bowel diseases (IBD), chronic ischemia, actinic proctitis, rectal neoformation, and in patients undergoing resection surgery of the rectum [32, 34, 54]. In this situation the calculated compliance is reduced.
- impaired evacuation and impaired rectal force during attempted defecation (push) in most patients with fecal incontinence, especially those with fecal seepage. They might be unable to expel the balloon from rectum in 2 min suggesting the presence of an underlying disorder of defecation, often associated with hyposensitivity [34, 65–67].

2. Chronic Constipation (CC)

There are three underlying pathophysiological mechanism of chronic constipation (CC) recognized from transit studies: CC with normal transit (NTC) where the subject has symptoms of constipation but colorectal transit time is normal, CC with slow-transit constipation (STC) with abnormally slow transit throughout the whole colorectum, and CC with outlet obstruction where transit is mainly delayed in the distal colorectum.

Using ARM 27–59% of patients with chronic constipation can be classified with functional defecation disorders or dyssynergic defecation (DD), which refers to the paradoxical contraction or inadequate relaxation of the pelvic floor attempted defecation; an overlap of dyssynergic defecation and irritable bowel syndrome-predominant constipation (IBS-C) is commonly present [44, 68, 69].

However, the ARM diagnosis of a functional defecation disorder has to be supported by the evidence of impaired evacuation by either BET or imaging, according to the Rome IV criteria.

Moreover, a diagnosis of a functional defecation disorder is a predictor of successful biofeedback outcome in constipated patients [5, 21, 70].

The manometric examination allows recognizing in CC patients:

- Impaired rectal sensation. Threshold for first sensation and desire to defecate can be higher in 60% of patients with DD and are associated with an impaired rectal sensation, generally an increased rectal compliance, with rectal hyposensitivity, indicative of an excessively lax (floppy) rectum; higher volumes of rectal distention are required to elicit perception also in patients with important dilatation of the rectum (megarectum) [8, 46, 64, 71]. Rectal hyposensitivity can predict a poor response to treatments such as biofeedback or surgery because it indicates a severe clinical phenotype [72]; however, it has been described an improvement of symptom [66, 73], especially during treatment with neuromodulation [13].
- A subgroup of patients with DD can have structural disorders found on evacuation proctography or magnetic resonance imaging [69].
- An absent rectoanal inhibitory reflex in adult is more often due to chronic constipation with megacolon [33]; however, a failure of reflexive IAS relaxation in ARM allows the diagnosis of congenital ganglia of the myenteric plexus, Hirschsprung's disease; most cases of Hirschsprung's disease are detected in childhood, while short segment Hirschsprung's disease can be present in adulthood [32, 52].
- Very often more than one abnormality can be found in the same patient and abnormal tests are common among healthy subjects without symptoms of CC. Thus, no test can stand alone in the evaluation of individual patients.

3. Chronic Proctalgia

Chronic or recurrent pain in the anal canal, rectum, and pelvis can be detected in 7–24% of the population and is associated with impaired quality of life and high health care costs [74]. After the exclusion of organic causes, ARM allows to evaluate the presence of functional anorectal pain disorders or sphincter hypertonicity.

Functional anorectal pain disorders include both proctalgia fugax and levator ani syndrome (LAS), characterized by recurrent pain localized to the anus or lower rectum without evidence of anorectal disease; the first is defined by Rome IV criteria [48] as recurrent episodes of midline anal pain, lasting from seconds to minutes, <20 min, unrelated to defecation, for at least 3 months, with absence of anorectal pain between episodes; in a small group of patients with severe proctalgia, there may be a myopathy of the IAS [18, 65]. The second is characterized by recurrent anorectal pain occurring in episodes lasting >20 min, worse when sitting than standing; the symptoms may also include a chronic sensation of rectal fullness, urge to defecate, and tenderness during traction on the puborectalis [18].

Etiology is poorly defined, but a chronic spasm in the striated muscles of pelvic floor is often thought to be the pathophysiological mechanism for most of them. However, DD has been recently reported to be relevant etiology, even for patients without constipation symptoms [74].

In a large randomized controlled trial biofeedback, electrogalvanic stimulation and massage were compared for the treatment of chronic proctalgia. Biofeedback showed a success rate of 85% in patients with evidence of tenderness in response to traction on levator ani muscle. This is a physical sign suggestive of striated muscle tension [74].

In patients with chronic proctalgia and a normal structural evaluation, DD may play a role beyond constipation; hence, in these patients ARM with BET should be employed early to diagnose DD. In fact, impaired pelvic floor muscle relaxation and abnormal BET have been shown to be related to anorectal pain and have a favorable response to biofeedback therapy [66].

4. Preoperative and postoperative evaluations of patients with anorectal disease

Candidates to ARM are patients with anorectal pathologies (prolapse, fissures, hemorrhoids, tumors) or with RCU in view of recanalization after Hartmann's intervention or to evaluate the feasibility of an ileo-anus-anastomosis. The comparison between the data detected by pre- and post-surgery manometry can provide useful information to interpret the causes of any disturbances or problems that have arisen or otherwise remained unchanged.

5. Finally, the role of manometry for *Legal Medical Purposes* should not be underestimated: the possibility of documenting what the intervention performed has modified in terms of rectal-anal functionality, might be supporting a negative diagnosis of procedure related symptoms.

6. Biofeedback Therapy (BFT)

The anorectal manometry contributes significantly to the recognition of defecation disorders or dyssynergic defecation (DD) and it provides the main indication for rehabilitation programs through the implementation of a biofeedback training for the recovery of anorectal and pelvic floor function [75].

This therapy is an "operant conditioning" technique, in which information about a physiological process (recorded by electromyographic sensors or manometry) is converted into a specific signal able to teach the patient to control a function. This allows to restore a normal pattern of defecation, correcting dyssynergia or incoordination of abdominal and pelvic floor muscles and anal sphincter, to obtain a normal and complete evacuation, and to improve perception in patients with impaired rectal sensation [20, 46, 55].

Moreover, patients can learn to expel an air filled balloon, and if reduced rectal sensation is present, they can learn to recognized weaker sensations of rectal filling, through sensory retraining [20]. Rehabilitation therapy may also include measures to improve pelvic floor contraction (i.e., Kegel exercises) [66].

BFT has 70–80% of efficacy in randomized controlled trials, more effective than diet or pharmacological therapy (polyethylene glycol or diazepam or placebo) [33, 66, 76–79].

Long-term studies have shown that its beneficial effect is maintained for more than 2 years after treatment [66, 80, 81], although important alteration of sensitivity and compliance have an unfavorable prognosis on BFT results.

BFT has been shown efficacy in about 76% of patients with FI [82] and is recommended when conservative management failed [83–85]. However, meta-analyses suggest that the efficacy of BFT in FI is still controversial [86]. It is widely accepted that a reduction in FI episodes/week by ≥50% can be considered a valid and clinical outcomes measure, and it correlates well with bowel symptoms and its severity [85–87].

3.5   Contraindications to Arm

Relative contraindications are the presence of bloody fissures and active proctitis of different etiology; in these cases the manometric procedure can exacerbate the pain and produce an important anorectal bleeding.

Absolute contraindications are represented by recent surgical interventions on the anorectal region, poor patient compliance to procedure, and severe anal stenosis.

3.6   Limitations of ARM

The interpretative difficulties of the results, due to wide variability and overlap of manometric measurements in health and disease, the discussed impact on the outcomes of patients, the high costs of dedicated equipment, strongly limit the use of anorectal manometry in clinical practice, as well as its widespread diffusion [3].

Moreover, the anorectal manometry is characterized by a certain intra- and inter-operator variability, both in the execution of the examination (given the considerable heterogeneity of the available instruments) and in the interpretation of the results.

The recent use of the new computerized technologies, the elaboration of standard execution protocols [17], and the publication of the normality limits of the manometric parametric principles [25, 26, 33, 88–90] have partly reduced intraoperator variability, contributing to the standardization of the anorectal manometry both in the executive and interpretative aspects.

3.6.1   High-Resolution Anorectal Manometry

Recently, an advanced high-resolution anorectal manometry (HRAM) (or high definition manometry—HDAM) has been introduced, providing a dedicated software and specific solid-state probe with sensors able to provide a detailed topographic and colorimetric mapping of the anorectal and a more intuitive evaluation of the anorectal function without the need for pull-through of the catheter [91, 92].

This new technique would be able to show in detail the various subgroups of patients with dyssynergic defecation and detect the defects of the anal sphincter at rest and during squeeze in great detail [44, 93].

HRAM is significantly more expensive and is more likely to be found at high-volume academic centers but allows interpretation of topographical plots of anorectal function. Conventional ARM allows an inexpensive screening test for community practitioners often requiring less space and staff support. Because of the significant differences in testing equipment available and interoperator differences in performance and interpretation of test, there is a large amount of heterogeneity in the results of ARM. Furthermore, the high costs of the technology still strongly limit its diffusion and therefore its use in clinical practice [33].

Use of HRAM seems to be more intuitive, showing a large amount of data into a detailed color topography. HRAM is very clever to stratify patients with DD into subgroups, and this could allow to incorporate the multiple parameters derived from HRAM into a classification scheme similar to the Chicago classification that has revolutionized the diagnosis of esophageal motility disorders [93, 94].

References

1. Palit S, Lunniss PJ, Scott SM. The physiology of human defecation. Dig Dis Sci. 2012;57(6):1445–64.
2. Perry S, Shaw C, McGrother C, Matthews RJ, Assassa RP, Dallosso H, et al. Prevalence of faecal incontinence in adults aged 40 years or more living in the community. Gut. 2002;50(4):480–4.
3. Carrington EV, Scott SM, Bharucha A, Mion F, Remes-Troche JM, Malcolm A, et al. Expert consensus document: advances in the evaluation of anorectal function. Nat Rev Gastroenterol Hepatol. 2018;15(5):309–23.
4. Neri L, Conway PM, Basilisco G, Laxative Inadequate Relief Survey (LIRS) Group. Confirmatory factor analysis of the Patient Assessment of Constipation-Symptoms (PAC-SYM) among patients with chronic constipation. Qual Life Res. 2015;24(7):1597–605.
5. Tantiphlachiva K, Rao P, Attaluri A, Rao SS. Digital rectal examination is a useful tool for identifying patients with dyssynergia. Clin Gastroenterol Hepatol. 2010;8(11):955–60.
6. Lam TJ, Felt-Bersma RJ. Clinical examination remains more important than anorectal function tests to identify treatable conditions in women with constipation. Int Urogynecol J. 2013;24(1):67–72.
7. Camilleri M, Talley NJ. Pathophysiology as a basis for understanding symptom complexes and therapeutic targets. Neurogastroenterol Motil. 2004;16(2):135–42.
8. Scott SM, Gladman MA. Manometric, sensorimotor, and neurophysiologic evaluation of anorectal function. Gastroenterol Clin N Am. 2008;37(3):511–38, vii.
9. Neri L, Iovino P, Laxative Inadequate Relief Survey (LIRS) Group. Bloating is associated with worse quality of life, treatment satisfaction, and treatment responsiveness among patients with constipation-predominant irritable bowel syndrome and functional constipation. Neurogastroenterol Motil. 2016;28(4):581–91.
10. Dinning PG, Carrington EV, Scott SM. The use of colonic and anorectal high-resolution manometry and its place in clinical work and in research. Neurogastroenterol Motil. 2015;27(12):1693–708.
11. Dinning PG, Carrington EV, Scott SM. Colonic and anorectal motility testing in the high-resolution era. Curr Opin Gastroenterol. 2016;32(1):44–8.
12. Altomare DF, Rinaldi M, Petrolino M, Ripetti V, Masin A, Ratto C, et al. Reliability of electrophysiologic anal tests in predicting the outcome of sacral nerve modulation for fecal incontinence. Dis Colon Rectum. 2004;47(6):853–7.
13. Knowles CH, Thin N, Gill K, Bhan C, Grimmer K, Lunniss PJ, et al. Prospective randomized double-blind study of temporary sacral nerve stimulation in patients with rectal evacuatory dysfunction and rectal hyposensitivity. Ann Surg. 2012;255(4):643–9.

14. Chiarioni G, Bassotti G, Stanganini S, Vantini I, Whitehead WE. Sensory retraining is key to bio-feedback therapy for formed stool fecal incontinence. Am J Gastroenterol. 2002;97(1):109–17.
15. Vaizey CJ, Kamm MA. Prospective assessment of the clinical value of anorectal investigations. Digestion. 2000;61(3):207–14.
16. Rao SS, Patel RS. How useful are manometric tests of anorectal function in the management of defecation disorders? Am J Gastroenterol. 1997;92(3):469–75.
17. Rao SS, Azpiroz F, Diamant N, Enck P, Tougas G, Wald A. Minimum standards of anorectal manometry. Neurogastroenterol Motil. 2002;14(5):553–9.
18. Diamant NE, Kamm MA, Wald A, Whitehead WE. AGA technical review on anorectal testing techniques. Gastroenterology. 1999;116(3):735–60.
19. Rao SS. Pathophysiology of adult fecal incontinence. Gastroenterology. 2004;126(1 Suppl 1):S14–22.
20. American Gastroenterological Association, Bharucha AE, Dorn SD, Lembo A, Pressman A. American Gastroenterological Association medical position statement on constipation. Gastroenterology. 2013;144(1):211–7.
21. Rao SS, Ozturk R, Laine L. Clinical utility of diagnostic tests for constipation in adults: a systematic review. Am J Gastroenterol. 2005;100(7):1605–15.
22. Bharucha AE, Rao SS. An update on anorectal disorders for gastroenterologists. Gastroenterology. 2014;146(1):37–45.e2.
23. Renzi A, Brillantino A, Di Sarno G, Izzo D, D'Aniello F, Falato A. Improved clinical outcomes with a new contour-curved stapler in the surgical treatment of obstructed defecation syndrome: a mid-term randomized controlled trial. Dis Colon Rectum. 2011;54(6):736–42.
24. Barnett JL, Hasler WL, Camilleri M. American Gastroenterological Association medical position statement on anorectal testing techniques. American Gastroenterological Association. Gastroenterology. 1999;116(3):732–60.
25. Gruppo Lombardo per lo Studio della Motilità Intestinale. Anorectal manometry with water-perfused catheter in healthy adults with no functional bowel disorders. Colorectal Dis. 2010;12(3):220–5.
26. Rao SS, Hatfield R, Soffer E, Rao S, Beaty J, Conklin JL. Manometric tests of anorectal function in healthy adults. Am J Gastroenterol. 1999;94(3):773–83.
27. Bordeianou LG, Carmichael JC, Paquette IM, Wexner S, Hull TL, Bernstein M, et al. Consensus statement of definitions for anorectal physiology testing and pelvic floor terminology (revised). Dis Colon Rectum. 2018;61(4):421–7.
28. Lestar B, Penninckx F, Kerremans R. The composition of anal basal pressure. An in vivo and in vitro study in man. Int J Color Dis. 1989;4(2):118–22.
29. Kim JH. How to interpret conventional anorectal manometry. J Neurogastroenterol Motil. 2010;16(4):437–9.
30. Videlock EJ, Lembo A, Cremonini F. Diagnostic testing for dyssynergic defecation in chronic constipation: meta-analysis. Neurogastroenterol Motil. 2013;25(6):509–20.
31. McHugh SM, Diamant NE. Effect of age, gender, and parity on anal canal pressures. Contribution of impaired anal sphincter function to fecal incontinence. Dig Dis Sci. 1987;32(7):726–36.
32. Chiou AW, Lin JK, Wang FM. Anorectal abnormalities in progressive systemic sclerosis. Dis Colon Rectum. 1989;32(5):417–21.
33. Staller K. Role of anorectal manometry in clinical practice. Curr Treat Options Gastroenterol. 2015;13(4):418–31.
34. Azpiroz F, Enck P, Whitehead WE. Anorectal functional testing: review of collective experience. Am J Gastroenterol. 2002;97(2):232–40.
35. Gladman MA, Dvorkin LS, Lunniss PJ, Williams NS, Scott SM. Rectal hyposensitivity: a disorder of the rectal wall or the afferent pathway? An assessment using the barostat. Am J Gastroenterol. 2005;100(1):106–14.
36. Gregersen H, Kassab G. Biomechanics of the gastrointestinal tract. Neurogastroenterol Motil. 1996;8(4):277–97.
37. Burgell RE, Scott SM. Rectal hyposensitivity. J Neurogastroenterol Motil. 2012;18(4):373–84.

38. Sun WM, Read NW, Prior A, Daly JA, Cheah SK, Grundy D. Sensory and motor responses to rectal distention vary according to rate and pattern of balloon inflation. Gastroenterology. 1990;99(4):1008–15.
39. Chan CL, Scott SM, Williams NS, Lunniss PJ. Rectal hypersensitivity worsens stool frequency, urgency, and lifestyle in patients with urge fecal incontinence. Dis Colon Rectum. 2005;48(1):134–40.
40. Iovino P, Valentini G, Ciacci C, De Luca A, Tremolaterra F, Sabbatini F, et al. Proximal stomach function in systemic sclerosis: relationship with autonomic nerve function. Dig Dis Sci. 2001;46(4):723–30.
41. Iovino P, Tremolaterra F, Boccia G, Miele E, Ruju FM, Staiano A. Irritable bowel syndrome in childhood: visceral hypersensitivity and psychosocial aspects. Neurogastroenterol Motil. 2009;21(9):940–e74.
42. Tremolaterra F, Gallotta S, Morra Y, Lubrano E, Ciacci C, Iovino P. The severity of irritable bowel syndrome or the presence of fibromyalgia influencing the perception of visceral and somatic stimuli. BMC Gastroenterol. 2014;14:182.
43. Bharucha AE, Pemberton JH, Locke GR 3rd. American Gastroenterological Association technical review on constipation. Gastroenterology. 2013;144(1):218–38.
44. Rao SS, Patcharatrakul T. Diagnosis and treatment of dyssynergic defecation. J Neurogastroenterol Motil. 2016;22(3):423–35.
45. Grossi U, Carrington EV, Bharucha AE, Horrocks EJ, Scott SM, Knowles CH. Diagnostic accuracy study of anorectal manometry for diagnosis of dyssynergic defecation. Gut. 2016;65(3):447–55.
46. Rao SS. Dyssynergic defecation and biofeedback therapy. Gastroenterol Clin N Am. 2008;37(3):569–86, viii.
47. Longstreth GF, Thompson WG, Chey WD, Houghton LA, Mearin F, Spiller RC. Functional bowel disorders. Gastroenterology. 2006;130(5):1480–91.
48. Mearin F, Lacy BE, Chang L, Chey WD, Lembo AJ, Simren M, et al. Bowel disorders. Gastroenterology. 2016. https://doi.org/10.1053/j.gastro.2016.02.031.
49. Chiarioni G, Kim SM, Vantini I, Whitehead WE. Validation of the balloon evacuation test: reproducibility and agreement with findings from anorectal manometry and electromyography. Clin Gastroenterol Hepatol. 2014;12(12):2049–54.
50. Gladman MA, Aziz Q, Scott SM, Williams NS, Lunniss PJ. Rectal hyposensitivity: pathophysiological mechanisms. Neurogastroenterol Motil. 2009;21(5):508–16, e4-5.
51. Kamm MA. Obstetric damage and faecal incontinence. Lancet. 1994;344(8924):730–3.
52. Engel AF, Kamm MA, Bartram CI, Nicholls RJ. Relationship of symptoms in faecal incontinence to specific sphincter abnormalities. Int J Color Dis. 1995;10(3):152–5.
53. Simren M, Tornblom H, Palsson OS, van Tilburg MAL, Van Oudenhove L, Tack J, et al. Visceral hypersensitivity is associated with GI symptom severity in functional GI disorders: consistent findings from five different patient cohorts. Gut. 2018;67(2):255–62.
54. Rao GN, Drew PJ, Lee PW, Monson JR, Duthie GS. Anterior resection syndrome is secondary to sympathetic denervation. Int J Color Dis. 1996;11(5):250–8.
55. Chiarioni G. Biofeedback treatment of chronic constipation: myths and misconceptions. Tech Coloproctol. 2016;20(9):611–8.
56. Bharucha AE. Fecal incontinence. Gastroenterology. 2003;124(6):1672–85.
57. Whitehead WE, Borrud L, Goode PS, Meikle S, Mueller ER, Tuteja A, et al. Fecal incontinence in US adults: epidemiology and risk factors. Gastroenterology. 2009;137(2):512–7, 517. e1-2
58. Rao SS. Advances in diagnostic assessment of fecal incontinence and dyssynergic defecation. Clin Gastroenterol Hepatol. 2010;8(11):910–9.
59. Vaizey CJ, Kamm MA, Bartram CI. Primary degeneration of the internal anal sphincter as a cause of passive faecal incontinence. Lancet. 1997;349(9052):612–5.
60. Felt-Bersma RJ, Klinkenberg-Knol EC, Meuwissen SG. Anorectal function investigations in incontinent and continent patients. Differences and discriminatory value. Dis Colon Rectum. 1990;33(6):479–85; discussion 85-6.

61. Chiarioni G, Scattolini C, Bonfante F, Vantini I. Liquid stool incontinence with severe urgency: anorectal function and effective biofeedback treatment. Gut. 1993;34(11):1576–80.
62. Sun WM, Donnelly TC, Read NW. Utility of a combined test of anorectal manometry, electromyography, and sensation in determining the mechanism of 'idiopathic' faecal incontinence. Gut. 1992;33(6):807–13.
63. Sangwan YP, Coller JA, Schoetz DJ, Roberts PL, Murray JJ. Spectrum of abnormal rectoanal reflex patterns in patients with fecal incontinence. Dis Colon Rectum. 1996;39(1):59–65.
64. Harraf F, Schmulson M, Saba L, Niazi N, Fass R, Munakata J, et al. Subtypes of constipation predominant irritable bowel syndrome based on rectal perception. Gut. 1998;43(3):388–94.
65. Rao SS, American College of Gastroenterology Practice Parameters Committee. Diagnosis and management of fecal incontinence. American College of Gastroenterology Practice Parameters Committee. Am J Gastroenterol. 2004;99(8):1585–604.
66. Chiarioni G, Whitehead WE, Pezza V, Morelli A, Bassotti G. Biofeedback is superior to laxatives for normal transit constipation due to pelvic floor dyssynergia. Gastroenterology. 2006;130(3):657–64.
67. Gladman MA, Scott SM, Chan CL, Williams NS, Lunniss PJ. Rectal hyposensitivity: prevalence and clinical impact in patients with intractable constipation and fecal incontinence. Dis Colon Rectum. 2003;46(2):238–46.
68. Patcharatrakul T, Gonlachanvit S. Outcome of biofeedback therapy in dyssynergic defecation patients with and without irritable bowel syndrome. J Clin Gastroenterol. 2011;45(7):593–8.
69. Krogh K, Chiarioni G, Whitehead W. Management of chronic constipation in adults. United European Gastroenterol J. 2017;5(4):465–72.
70. Rao SS. Constipation: evaluation and treatment. Gastroenterol Clin N Am. 2003;32(2):659–83.
71. Gladman MA, Knowles CH. Novel concepts in the diagnosis, pathophysiology and management of idiopathic megabowel. Colorectal Dis. 2008;10(6):531–8; discussion 8-40.
72. Rhee PL, Choi MS, Kim YH, Son HJ, Kim JJ, Koh KC, et al. An increased rectal maximum tolerable volume and long anal canal are associated with poor short-term response to biofeedback therapy for patients with anismus with decreased bowel frequency and normal colonic transit time. Dis Colon Rectum. 2000;43(10):1405–11.
73. Rao SS, Welcher KD, Pelsang RE. Effects of biofeedback therapy on anorectal function in obstructive defecation. Dig Dis Sci. 1997;42(11):2197–205.
74. Chiarioni G, Asteria C, Whitehead WE. Chronic proctalgia and chronic pelvic pain syndromes: new etiologic insights and treatment options. World J Gastroenterol. 2011;17(40):4447–55.
75. Chiarioni G, Heymen S, Whitehead WE. Biofeedback therapy for dyssynergic defecation. World J Gastroenterol. 2006;12(44):7069–74.
76. Heymen S, Scarlett Y, Jones K, Ringel Y, Drossman D, Whitehead WE. Randomized, controlled trial shows biofeedback to be superior to alternative treatments for patients with pelvic floor dyssynergia-type constipation. Dis Colon Rectum. 2007;50(4):428–41.
77. Rao SS, Valestin J, Brown CK, Zimmerman B, Schulze K. Long-term efficacy of biofeedback therapy for dyssynergic defecation: randomized controlled trial. Am J Gastroenterol. 2010;105(4):890–6.
78. Payne I, Grimm LM Jr. Functional disorders of constipation: paradoxical puborectalis contraction and increased perineal descent. Clin Colon Rectal Surg. 2017;30(1):22–9.
79. Jodorkovsky D, Dunbar KB, Gearhart SL, Stein EM, Clarke JO. Biofeedback therapy for defecatory dysfunction: "real life" experience. J Clin Gastroenterol. 2013;47(3):252–5.
80. Rao SS, Seaton K, Miller M, Brown K, Nygaard I, Stumbo P, et al. Randomized controlled trial of biofeedback, sham feedback, and standard therapy for dyssynergic defecation. Clin Gastroenterol Hepatol. 2007;5(3):331–8.
81. Lee HJ, Boo SJ, Jung KW, Han S, Seo SY, Koo HS, et al. Long-term efficacy of biofeedback therapy in patients with dyssynergic defecation: results of a median 44 months follow-up. Neurogastroenterol Motil. 2015;27(6):787–95.

82. Rao SS, Welcher KD, Happel J. Can biofeedback therapy improve anorectal function in fecal incontinence? Am J Gastroenterol. 1996;91(11):2360–6.
83. Enck P, Daublin G, Lubke HJ, Strohmeyer G. Long-term efficacy of biofeedback training for fecal incontinence. Dis Colon Rectum. 1994;37(10):997–1001.
84. Ozturk R, Niazi S, Stessman M, Rao SS. Long-term outcome and objective changes of anorectal function after biofeedback therapy for faecal incontinence. Aliment Pharmacol Ther. 2004;20(6):667–74.
85. Rao SS, Benninga MA, Bharucha AE, Chiarioni G, Di Lorenzo C, Whitehead WE. ANMS-ESNM position paper and consensus guidelines on biofeedback therapy for anorectal disorders. Neurogastroenterol Motil. 2015;27(5):594–609.
86. Rao SS. Endpoints for therapeutic interventions in faecal incontinence: small step or game changer. Neurogastroenterol Motil. 2016;28(8):1123–33.
87. Noelting J, Zinsmeister AR, Bharucha AE. Validating endpoints for therapeutic trials in fecal incontinence. Neurogastroenterol Motil. 2016;28(8):1148–56.
88. Sun WM, Rao SS. Manometric assessment of anorectal function. Gastroenterol Clin N Am. 2001;30(1):15–32.
89. Carrington EV, Grossi U, Knowles CH, Scott SM. Normal values for high-resolution anorectal manometry: a time for consensus and collaboration. Neurogastroenterol Motil. 2014;26(9):1356–7.
90. Li Y, Yang X, Xu C, Zhang Y, Zhang X. Normal values and pressure morphology for three-dimensional high-resolution anorectal manometry of asymptomatic adults: a study in 110 subjects. Int J Color Dis. 2013;28(8):1161–8.
91. Lee YY, Erdogan A, Rao SS. High resolution and high definition anorectal manometry and pressure topography: diagnostic advance or a new kid on the block? Curr Gastroenterol Rep. 2013;15(12):360.
92. Rao SS, Hasler WL. Can high-resolution anorectal manometry shed new light on defecatory disorders? Gastroenterology. 2013;144(2):263–5.
93. Ratuapli SK, Bharucha AE, Noelting J, Harvey DM, Zinsmeister AR. Phenotypic identification and classification of functional defecatory disorders using high-resolution anorectal manometry. Gastroenterology. 2013;144(2):314–22.e2.
94. Kahrilas PJ, Bredenoord AJ, Fox M, Gyawali CP, Roman S, Smout AJ, et al. The Chicago Classification of esophageal motility disorders, v3.0. Neurogastroenterol Motil. 2015;27(2):160–74.

Concept and Development of HRM: The Way It Works

4

Irene Martinucci, Nicola de Bortoli, Santino Marchi, and Dario Gambaccini

The study of gastrointestinal motility is essential for the diagnosis of some digestive diseases. However, direct evaluation of the effective muscle contraction (for example with electromyography) would be impossible. For this reason, today we base the study of motility on an indirect method, the manometry. This latter plans to evaluate the contraction by recording the pressure offered by the closure of the intestinal lumen against a catheter, as a function of time. The recording of the pressure variations allows therefore to evaluate the propagation of peristalsis or the presence of relaxation of the sphincter apparatus. For this reason, systems for the recording of intraluminal pressure events have evolved over the years from simple balloons to perfused and solid-state catheters. At the same time, display and analysis methods have evolved from strip chart recorders to computerized systems. Each advance has led to a better understanding of the pathophysiological mechanisms and therefore to a more accurate diagnosis of gastrointestinal motor disorders. More generally, manometric systems transmit data through catheters containing pressure sensors. The pressure sensors capture intraluminal pressure signals and transfer them to a receiving device, which records and displays data. Conventional measurements involve a set of two-dimensional tracings, the size of the set being determined by the number of recording ports or transducers located on the intraluminal probe [1–3]. The first manometric systems allowed recording on average of eight pressure sensors. The typical esophageal catheter included 4 radial channels for the evaluation of the lower esophageal sphincter and 4 sensors positioned at 5 cm distance from each other, to evaluate the peristaltic wave propagation. The typical anorectal

I. Martinucci
Gastrointestinal Unit, Versilia Hospital, Lido di Camaiore, Italy

N. de Bortoli · S. Marchi
Gastrointestinal Unit, Department of Translational Research and New Technologies in Medicine and Surgery, University of Pisa, Pisa, Italy

D. Gambaccini (✉)
Unit of Interventional and Pediatric Endoscopy, Cisanello Hospital, Pisa, Italy

© Springer Nature Switzerland AG 2020
M. Bellini (ed.), *High Resolution and High Definition Anorectal Manometry*,
https://doi.org/10.1007/978-3-030-32419-3_4

catheter, on the other hand, usually included eight pressure channels, but placed at 0.5 cm from each other, often also in a spiral shape. The low cost of perfused catheters also permitted for customization, such as the Dent sleeve catheter, which allowed for a better evaluation of the lower esophageal sphincter. However, these catheters admitted only the visualization of a 2D wave pattern, which required an adequate and longer training for its interpretation.

The first attempts to change the normal visualization of the manometric record were performed on the esophageal manometry [1, 2, 6]. In the 1990s Ray Eugene Clouse conceived and realized two significant advances of conventional manometric techniques: an increase in pressure sensors along the catheter, and the use of spatiotemporal plots for data display [4, 5].

At the beginning Clouse and Staiano hypothesized that spatial relationships of intraluminal pressure events, detected with manometric catheter, from one esophageal level to another, were not easily understood using a conventional strip chart recorder, particularly if the recording pressure sensors are spaced several centimeters apart along the esophageal length [1, 4]. They tested this hypothesis by continuing the pull-through maneuver 1 cm at a time till the last recording channels reached the upper esophageal sphincter, obtaining at least one wet swallows at each station. Then, a computerized topographic plotting system was employed to subsequently determine the spatial relationship of waves from each esophageal level. In this way, they demonstrated previously unrecognized wave relationships [1]. These results supported the idea that individual swallows could be studied with the topographic method using probes that have closely spaced recording sites.

The first methods of translating the manometric signal into an image were extremely cumbersome and not very intuitive. However, Clouse et al. [1, 2, 4, 6] developed a method of topographic analysis enabling to consider and evaluate time, spatial relations, and pressure data at the same time. This innovative intuition supported the hypothesis that more information could be extracted by considering spatial relationships of pressure data with a system able to record esophageal pressure from up to 21 sites and using two- and three-dimensional plotting methods. The first step in topographic representation was to align the recorded pressure data on a planar surface, with recording sites disposed on z-axis in accordance with their positions on the catheter. Time in seconds, after the event marker, is represented on x and amplitude of pressure (mmHg) on y. The y values (pressure amplitude) are interpolated using available neighboring data at each grid intersection so it is possible to establish the most appropriate value. In this way it is possible to obtain a single "overhead" perspective of three-dimensional measurements as weather or geographic data are commonly displayed. Figure 4.1 shows 9 traces as displayed by conventional methods (a) and by the corresponding planar representation (b) [7]. The second step was to apply time and pressure contour lines to the tracings with isobaric pressure lines (conventionally with intervals of 5-mmHg) (Fig. 4.2a). The colors are linked to pressures to form a progressive color profile plot: cooler colors for lower pressures and warmer colors for higher pressures. With the contour plots it is possible to have an overhead perspective of surface plots, with contour ring encompassing the specific amplitudes with a specific color. Concentric rings

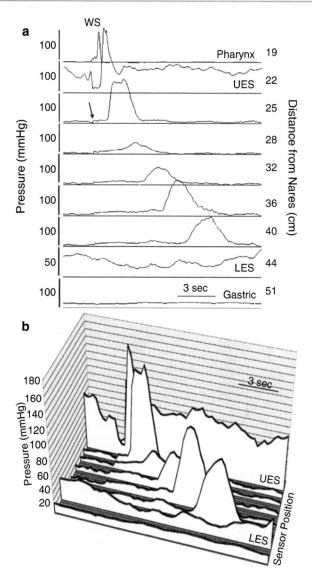

Fig. 4.1 In the conventional manometry intraluminal pressures are recorded from widely spaced sensors (3- to 5-cm). (**a**) In this two-dimensional display pressure is on the *y*-axis, time is on the *x*-axis, and pressure tracings are stacked vertically. (**b**) Tracings are displayed three-dimensionally: pressure remains on the *y*-axis and time on the *x*-axis but sensor position is on the z-axis with the gastric sensor at the front and the pharynx sensor at the back

indicate a regional pressure peak on the plot. In this system it is also possible to shift the plot baseline choosing the zero on the point of interest (e.g., in esophageal manometry to mark intragastric pressure). Initially, surface plots were more easily interpreted because conventional wave forms could be recognized within the

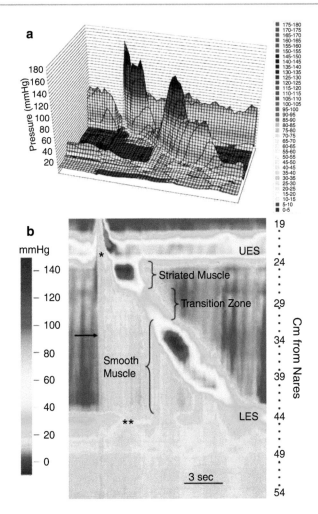

Fig. 4.2 (**a**) Application of pressure contour lines with isobaric pressure lines (5-mmHg). Colors are linked to a specific color profile plot: cooler colors for lower pressures and warmer colors for higher pressures. (**b**) Esophageal manometry: The definitive and commonly used display obtained by rotating plot until the direction of eyes is parallel to *y*-axis. Pressure axis (*y*) collapses and it is replaced by a color contour for a handier two-dimensional surface

three-dimensional structures. However, once the investigators became familiar with viewing and interpreting contour plots, this format proved significant advantages over surface plots including: the possibility to measure characteristics of peristalsis in specific regions of interest without concern of possible interferences with the three-dimensional perspective; the ability to see all the pressure data in their entirety and complexity, without losing information that might be obscured from view in the three-dimensional surface plots and making easier direct inter-swallow and inter-subject comparisons [8, 9]. As a result, a topographic analysis system was thus available for studying time and space relationships of pressure data, being helpful in displaying the large amount of data and eliminating the burden that would otherwise result from the cumbersome data set.

Using such a novel computerized plotting method, the pressure changes are viewed from clinically useful and visually attractive three-dimensional graphic displays rather than as a series of isolated waves [9, 10]. Considerations of both time and space relationships of pressure data acquired from intraluminal recording have revealed more accurate information regarding the direction of the wave movement, and the evaluation of all pressure events occurring over a length of studied organ has revealed more information about the neuromuscular mechanisms involved in local motility [10]. Moreover, the developed system requires no manipulation or summation of the pressure data, thus enabling to determine abnormalities identified in isolated time windows that may not be occurring "on the average," and provides a simplified and rapid method of analyzing pressure data from several visual perspectives.

Overall, with the advent of high-resolution manometry, the pressure sensors are closely spaced, and the overall number of pressure sensors is increased. With these modifications, much more information can be acquired, as data are not lost in the gaps that are typically present in a conventional catheter, which typically has 4–8 pressure sensors placed 3–5 cm of each other. Moreover, this novel technology provides color-countered topographic plots based on amplitude, distance, and time, depicting a continuum of dynamic pressure changes along lengths and time; data are presented in a simplified manner, in contrast to the use of linear plots of amplitude signals alone in conventional manometry.

Over time, the most intuitive visualization, that is commonly used today during manometric examinations, has become more and more established. This kind of visualization (Fig. 4.2b) has been obtained by rotating plot so that the operator looks down on it from directly above, with the direction of his/her eyes parallel to y-axis. In this way the pressure axis (y) breaks down and instead of a three-dimensional color contour we obtain a handier two-dimensional surface in which pressure is represented by colors. At this point sensor location is on the y-axis, and time is on the x-axis [7]. These novel techniques have already proven useful in both research and clinical settings, giving greater insight into normal and abnormal motor function than conventional manometric methods [11].

Although these measurement and analysis methods were first used in the esophagus, they are applicable in other parts of the gastrointestinal tract. High-resolution anorectal manometry (HRAM) was introduced in 2008, followed by high-definition anorectal manometry (HDAM), to achieve more precise measurements of anorectal pressure using densely arranged catheter sensors, and thus, to improve our diagnostic yield for anorectal disorders [12–14]. Indeed, whereas the conventional catheters have 4–8 unidirectional sensors, HRAM or HDAM catheters have multiple pressure sensors that straddle the entire anal canal and more proximal sensors inside a balloon placed in the rectum. Therefore, HRAM and HDAM catheters provide better spatial resolution of the sphincter pressure profile than conventional catheters. Station pull-through maneuvers are not required, which minimize movement related

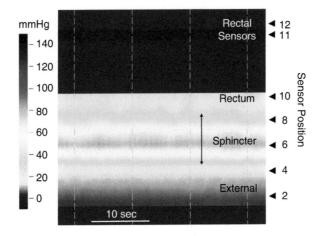

Fig. 4.3 Resting anorectal motor function. Different colors correspond to different pressure as reported on the color-pressure scale on the left. Sensor location is on the *y*-axis and time is on the *x*-axis

artifacts and shorten the procedure duration (Fig. 4.3) [7]. Furthermore, even if a contraction can occur with an upward displacement (e.g., during bearing down), the spatial resolution of the catheter allows the register also this event, providing more information. Also, there is now the theoretical possibility to test patient in the defecatory position, permitting new insights in a more physiological way.

Despite the advantages brought by the high definition, there are still limits of the method that will be dealt with in detail in the next chapters in order to rigorously evaluate the incremental clinical utility of HRAM or HDAM compared to non-high resolution manometry.

References

1. Clouse RE, Staiano A, Alrakawi A. Development of a topographic analysis system for manometric studies in the gastrointestinal tract. Gastrointest Endosc. 1998;48(4):395–401.
2. Clouse RE, Staiano A, Alrakawi A, Haroian L. Application of topographical methods to clinical esophageal manometry. Am J Gastroenterol. 2000;95(10):2720–30.
3. Yadlapati R. High resolution manometry vs conventional line tracing for esophageal motility disorders. Gastroenterol Hepatol (N Y). 2017;13(3):176–8.
4. Clouse RE, Staiano A. Topography of the esophageal peristaltic pressure wave. Am J Phys. 1991;261(4 Pt 1):G677–84.
5. Gyawali CP. High resolution manometry: the Ray Clouse legacy. Neurogastroenterol Motil. 2012;24(Suppl 1):2–4. https://doi.org/10.1111/j.1365-2982.2011.01836.x.
6. Clouse RE, Prakash C. Topographic esophageal manometry: an emerging clinical and investigative approach. Dig Dis. 2000;18(2):64–74.
7. Conklin J, Pimentel M, Soffer EE. Color atlas of high resolution manometry. New York: Springer; 2009. https://doi.org/10.1007/978-0-387-88295-6.
8. Dhawan I, O'Connell B, Patel A, Schey R, Parkman HP, Friedenberg F. Utility of esophageal high-resolution manometry in clinical practice: first, do HRM. Dig Dis Sci. 2018;63(12):3178–86. https://doi.org/10.1007/s10620-018-5300-4.

9. Keller J. What is the impact of high-resolution manometry in the functional diagnostic workup of gastroesophageal reflux disease? Visc Med. 2018;34(2):101–8. https://doi.org/10.1159/000486883.
10. Gyawali CP, de Bortoli N, Clarke J, Marinelli C, Tolone S, Roman S, Savarino E. Indications and interpretation of esophageal function testing. Ann N Y Acad Sci. 2018;1434(1):239–53. https://doi.org/10.1111/nyas.13709.
11. Kahrilas PJ, Bredenoord AJ, Carlson DA, Pandolfino JE. Advances in management of esophageal motility disorders. Clin Gastroenterol Hepatol. 2018;16(11):1692–700. https://doi.org/10.1016/j.cgh.2018.04.026.
12. Lee YY, Erdogan A, Rao SS. High resolution and high definition anorectal manometry and pressure topography: diagnostic advance or a new kid on the block? Curr Gastroenterol Rep. 2013;15(12):360. https://doi.org/10.1007/s11894-013-0360-2.
13. Lee TH, Bharucha AE. How to perform and interpret a high-resolution anorectal manometry test. J Neurogastroenterol Motil. 2016;22(1):46–59. https://doi.org/10.5056/jnm15168.
14. Jones MP, Post J, Crowell MD. High-resolution manometry in the evaluation of anorectal disorders: a simultaneous comparison with water-perfused manometry. Am J Gastroenterol. 2007;102(4):850–5.

Differences Between Conventional Anorectal Manometry and High Resolution/High Definition Anorectal Manometry

5

Francesco Torresan, Daniele Mandolesi,
Sebastiano Bonventre, and Paolo Usai-Satta

5.1   Conventional Anorectal Manometry and Its Limits

During the last 20 years many studies investigated and discussed the usefulness of manometry in studying anorectal function and dysfunctions. Conventional anorectal manometry (ARM) measures anal canal pressures in static and dynamic conditions and is traditionally considered a valuable test for the diagnosis and management of anorectal disorders.

ARM is the best diagnostic tool able to provide a direct assessment of anal sphincter pressure and rectoanal response during squeezing and straining maneuvers. Unfortunately, each motility laboratory performs ARM in a different way with different manners of reporting results and conclusions.

Perfusion catheters are generally employed because solid-state microtransducers, which are more reliable, are considered to be too expensive for routine use. ARM, together with other functional tests, can provide essential information on the anorectal pathophysiology of defecation disturbances such as functional defecation disorders and fecal incontinence (FI).

The biggest pitfall of conventional ARM is the lack of uniformity regarding equipment and technique: indeed no consensus was definitely reached about the optimal method for performing an anorectal manometric assessment using conventional systems [1] and the interpretation of ARM findings can be difficult

F. Torresan (✉) · D. Mandolesi
Department of Medical and Surgical Sciences, Policlinico Sant'Orsola Malpighi,
Bologna, Italy
e-mail: francesco.torresan@aosp.bo.it

S. Bonventre
Department of Surgical, Oncological and Oral Science, University of Palermo, Policlinico
P. Giaccone, Palermo, Italy

P. Usai-Satta
Gastroenterology Unit, G. Brotzu Hospital, Cagliari, Italy

© Springer Nature Switzerland AG 2020
M. Bellini (ed.), *High Resolution and High Definition Anorectal Manometry*,
https://doi.org/10.1007/978-3-030-32419-3_5

owing to the wide variability of the "normal values" among different laboratories [2]. Moreover, most of the parameters measured by ARM (i.e., anal canal pressure, sensory thresholds, etc.) are influenced not only by sex and age, but also by the protocol used.

Indeed normal anal canal pressures largely vary according to sex and age. In general, pressures are higher in men and younger subjects, but there is a considerable overlap between healthy subjects and patients. In addition, till now, most studies did not include large numbers of healthy subjects, consequently the age and sex-specific normal ranges used by the different motility laboratories are derived from the observation of small groups and they probably should be better standardized on larger samples. Due to these reasons some studies suggest that ARM would be able to offer only little additional utility over digital rectal examination for patients' management [3]. Moreover, ARM is relatively time consuming and its reliability depends on the operator's experience. All these problems limit a more widespread perception of its usefulness, and therefore its larger diffusion.

When performing ARM a potential risk of both false positive and false negative results should be considered since both patient's and catheter's position can affect objective measurements, especially in water-perfused ARM, where the probe is often repositioned during the different phases of the exam. Moreover pelvic floor abnormalities, such as pelvic floor descent and intra-anal intussusception, able to affect the results, are not reliably detected by ARM.

Despite these problems, the reproducibility of ARM is reported good. Hallan et al. [4] assessed anal sphincter function by digital examination and anal canal manometry in 66 patients and controls. They found a good correlation between digital basal score and maximum basal pressure (Spearman rank correlation coefficient rs = 0.56, $p < 0.001$). There were wide ranges of sphincter function on digital and manometric assessment with considerable overlap between patient groups. Another study showed that individual variation of resting pressures measured on two separate days was ≤12% indicating a good correlation between the two evaluations [5].

Quantitative measurements of ARM include resting pressure, automatic functions (e.g., rectoanal inhibitory reflex), and voluntary functions (i.e., squeeze pressure, anal relaxation and rectoanal pressure gradient during simulated defecation). Measurements of voluntary functions, requiring active participation by the patient, can vary with patient understanding of instructions. A recent study [6] showed that maximum squeeze pressure, intrarectal pressure, and rectoanal pressure gradient during the push maneuver were all significantly increased when "enhanced" verbal feedback was given to the patients, compared to the results from the same individuals when only "standard" instructions were provided. Such verbal intervention was able to change manometric findings from locally validated as "pathological" to "normal" in 14/31 patients (45%) with fecal incontinence and 12/39 (31%) with functional defecation disorders (Fig. 5.1). Indeed, an effective explanation of the procedures is required during the entire examination.

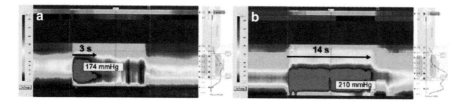

Fig. 5.1 Representative HRAM pressure topography plots of squeeze during standard (**a**) vs enhanced (**b**) instruction and verbal feedback, demonstrating increased pressure and prolongation of squeeze duration (black arrow) (reproduced from Heinrich et al. [6])

5.1.1 Sphincter Resting Pressure

Resting pressure is the result of the activity of the internal anal sphincter (IAS) and the external anal sphincter (EAS). Anal resting pressure is not uniform over the longitudinal extent of the anal canal. Conventional ARM catheters have a limited number of unidirectional sensors (up to eight) which often do not measure pressures over the entire length of the anal canal at the same time; moreover the measurement of resting pressure may be influenced by the ultraslow wave cycling activity [7].

5.1.2 Squeeze Pressure

The squeeze anal pressure measures voluntary contraction of the EAS. The squeeze pressure is lower in women than in men and lower in older than in younger people. Because ARM cannot assess contractile symmetry, it is not useful for identifying contraction of the puborectalis muscle, which only generates forces on the posterior side of the anorectal region; thus it is not able to assess if possible pressure changes are due to EAS or to a puborectalis muscle injury.

5.1.3 Straining Maneuver

During simulated evacuation, patients are asked to expel the manometric probe, typically with the balloon empty and less frequently with the balloon inflated with low air volumes. The assessment of pressure changes during simulated evacuation is limited by the type of recording catheter, the distension of the intrarectal balloon, the body position, the possible displacement of the catheter, and the degree of voluntary participation, because some people find it embarrassing to defecate in the laboratory without the necessary privacy. Finally, about 20% of asymptomatic healthy people undergoing ARM have manometric abnormalities characterizing a straining disorder [8].

5.1.4   Rectoanal Inhibitory Reflex (RAIR)

Rapid rectal distension by inflating the intrarectal balloon elicits an intrinsic reflex, mediated by the myenteric plexus, that relaxes the IAS. The absence of the intrinsic reflex during the rapid rectal distension is typical of the Hirschsprung disease so ARM proved to be a reliable and minimally invasive technique for the diagnosis of this disturbance.

In patients with acquired megarectum, RAIR may be absent because the rectal balloon does not adequately distend the rectum: in this case higher inflation volumes are able to elicit RAIR and therefore should be used in order to distinguish acquired megarectum from Hirschsprung disease.

ARM can also have a role to evaluate the persistance of sympotoms after surgery of Hirschsprung disease, although often it does not give enough information for understanding the cause of a possible persistence of obstructive symptoms [9].

5.1.5   Rectal Compliance and Sensation

Assessing rectal sensation involves the measurement of the volume able to evoke the so-called "first sensation" and subsequently urgency and maximum tolerable volume. The rectal balloons supplied with ARM catheters are usually relatively stiff and moreover their stiffness can vary over time in case of multiuse catheters which are cleaned and reused. For these reasons, rectal compliance and pressure thresholds for rectal sensation sometimes cannot be reliably measured with ARM. Particularly rectal compliance can be reliably assessed only using the barostat which is provided with a long infinitely compliant polyethylene bag [10].

5.1.5.1 Conventional ARM Versus High Resolution Anorectal Manometry

The introduction of 2D high resolution anorectal manometry (HRAM) system, acquiring measurements from at least ten closely spaced pressure sensors across the anal sphincter, removes the need for a pull-through procedure and provides visual feedback to the operator allowing maintenance of a stable catheter position. Both HRAM and 3D high resolution anorectal manometry (HDAM) offer a standardized technique during the examination, evaluating the same parameters for every patient. Unfortunately, we are still far from having a "Chicago classification" for HRAM/ HDAM, due to the lack of reliable normal values able to give a real homogeneity to the anorectal manometric reports and making them easily comparable.

Jones et al. [11] reported that HRAM values are highly correlated with water-perfused manometry measurements. In 29 patients resting, squeeze, and relaxation pressures were simultaneously recorded showing the two methods were significantly correlated although anal sphincter pressures recorded by HRAM tended to be higher than those recorded with conventional water-perfused ARM. Furthermore, HRAM provided greater resolution of the intraluminal pressure.

Ambartsumyan et al. studied 30 children with constipation showing that HDAM, compared to ARM, allowed to distinguish the individual contribution of each component of the intra-anal pressure [12]. In addition to these findings, HDAM could have the ability to better detect the normal asymmetry of pressures within the anal canal, with higher pressures in the posterior proximal and anterior distal regions of the sphincter.

A more recent study [13] performed in 14 patients showed that the ARM and HRAM were similar in misuring resting and squeezing pressures. It confeme that the measurement time for HRAM was significantly shorter than the one for conventional water-perfused ARM. Furthermore, some evidence support the hypothesis that pelvic floor abnormalities, not previously identified by conventional ARM, can be detected using HRAM.

5.1.5.2 HDAM Versus HRAM

HDAM utilizes a rigid probe made by 256 pressures sensors arranged in a 16×16 grid (i.e., 16 rows spaced 4 mm apart, each containing 16 circumferentially oriented sensors 2.1 mm apart) with an active area of measurement of 6.4 cm. This technology defines the anatomical anal morphology more precisely than HRAM. Manometric data undergo linear interpolation through dedicated software which displays 2D or 3D cylindrical topographical models of the anal canal which can be rotated and viewed from all sides.

Raja et al. [14] studied 231 consecutive patients to investigate the diagnostic utility of HDAM compared to HRAM. HDAM and HRAM studies performed from April 2012 to October 2013 were identified and re-interpreted by two blinded investigators. Disagreements were resolved by a third investigator. Puborectalis muscle (PR) visualization, focal defects of anal canal, and dyssynergy were reported. With HDAM, PR function was visualized in 81% (at rest), 97% (during squeeze), and 73% (during strain). PR was visualized less often at rest in FI than in constipated patients (68 vs. 85%, $p = 0.007$). Focal defects were identified twice as often in FI than in constipated patients (19 vs. 10%, $p = 0.113$). Twenty-nine defects (86% anterior) were visualized on HDAM. Inter-reader agreement between HRAM and HDAM was moderate for PR function ($\kappa = 0.471$), but fair for focal defects ($\kappa = 0.304$). (Figs. 5.2 and 5.3). This study suggests that HDAM provides additional information about structure and function of the anorectum undetectable through HRAM analysis alone.

5.2   Clinical Meaning of HRAM/HDAM

Up to now, the principal indications of HRAM and HDAM are the same of conventional ARM: e.g., the diagnostic workup of FI, chronic constipation, and Hirschsprung disease. They may be also used to improve the results of the pelvic rehabilitation training, assessing patients before the therapy, and/or objectively evaluating them when the rehabilitation course is completed.

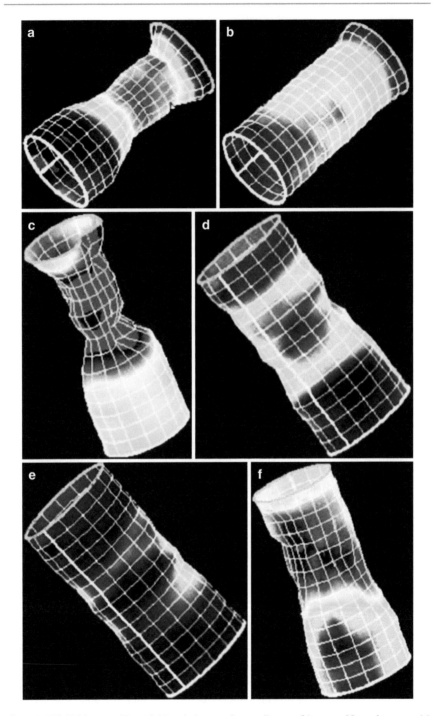

Fig. 5.2 HDAM images. Normal (**a**) and absent puborectalis tone (**b**) at rest. Normal squeeze (**c**) and focal defect at squeeze (**d**). Normal bear down (**e**) and paradoxical contraction (**f**) on bear down (reproduced from Raja et al. [14])

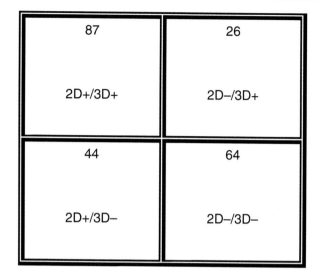

87	26
2D+/3D+	2D−/3D+
44	64
2D+/3D−	2D−/3D−

Fig. 5.3 2 × 2 Table for concordance between 2D and 3D diagnosis of dyssynergia. The + sign indicates the presence of dyssynergia respectively with 2D and 3D analysis (reproduced from Raja et al. [14])

5.2.1 Fecal Incontinence

FI is defined as the recurrent uncontrolled passage of fecal material for at least 3 months and is reported to affect 5–10% of the general population, affecting the quality of life and often leading to surgery [15, 16].

There is general agreement that the anal sphincter mechanism is the most important barrier against leakage of rectal contents [17].

Recent studies showed that anal resting and squeeze pressures measured with ARM and HDAM were lower in incontinent patients than in healthy persons.

Mion et al. conducted a prospective multicenter study in three groups of subjects: healthy asymptomatic controls, patients with FI, and patients with chronic constipation (CC) to evaluate how HDAM could differentiate patients with FI or CC from asymptomatic subjects. To distinguish FI from asymptomatic women, the two most important discriminant variables were: squeeze pressure (AUC of ROC: 0.786) and maximal squeeze pressure (AUC of ROC: 0.777) [18]. Push maneuver results were similar in the three groups, except for the nadir anal pressure that was significantly lower in FI women. Rectal constant defecatory sensation and maximum tolerable volumes were significantly lower in the FI women, compared to asymptomatic and CC women.

HDAM analysis of 24 asymptomatic healthy subjects and 24 patients with FI symptoms was performed; the authors developed and evaluated a robust prediction model to distinguish patients with FI from controls using linear discriminant, quadratic discriminant, and logistic regression analyses. FI severity index scores correlated with low resting pressure ($r = 0.34$) and peak squeeze pressure of the anal canal ($r = 0.28$). The combination of pressure values, anal sphincter area, and reflective symmetry values differentiated FI patients and controls with good accuracy (AUC: 0.96) [13]. Since the anal canal pressure is not symmetric along its length and circumference [19] and HDAM is able to better detect the length and the asymmetry of anal canal pressure [20–22], it appears particularly suitable for studying FI patients.

Finally, in a recent study on healthy women and women with FI, the use of a newly developed parameter, the HRAM contractile integral, increased the sensitivity of detection of anal hypocontractility, from 32% to 55%, compared with ARM measurements of squeeze [23].

5.2.2 Chronic Constipation

CC is a polysymptomatic, multifactorial disorder affecting 15–20% of the general population. It is characterized by symptoms of difficult, infrequent, or incomplete defecation. Lumpy or hard stools, sensation of anorectal obstruction/blockage, and manual maneuvers to facilitate the defecation are frequently reported [24].

A consistent number of patients with CC and irritable bowel syndrome with constipation also report symptoms suggestive of a functional defecation disorder (FDD) [25, 26], which is characterized by a paradoxical contraction or an inadequate relaxation of the pelvic floor muscles and/or inadequate propulsive forces during attempted defecation [27]. From a clinical point of view, FDD is frequently associated with excessive straining, feeling of incomplete evacuation, and digital facilitation of bowel movements [28]. However, symptoms do not consistently identify patients with FDD [29, 30]. Thus, the criteria for FDD must rely on both symptoms and physiological testing. Indeed, to diagnose FDD the Rome IV criteria require features of impaired evacuation in at least two of the following tests: anorectal manometry, rectal balloon expulsion test, barium or magnetic resonance (MR), defecography, and anal surface electromyography [27].

Manometric criteria for FDD include impaired anal relaxation, failure to increase rectal pressure, and a negative rectoanal gradient (i.e., rectal pressure lower than anal pressure) during simulated evacuation. However, Mion et al. [18] observed that many asymptomatic healthy people have a negative rectoanal gradient during evacuation, perhaps due to the left lateral position of the subjects during the procedure. Moreover, unlike normal defecation, during anorectal manometry the urge to defecate induced by rectal distention is not preceded by a normal predefecatory motor pattern associated with anal relaxation. Furthermore, patients may not completely understand the instructions provided during the test or may not be keen to accomplish the task [6, 31, 32].

From a manometric point of view, patients with FDD exhibit one of the following four abnormal defecation patterns [29] (Fig. 5.4):

- In type I the patient can generate adequate propulsive forces (rise in intrarectal pressure ≥ 40 mmHg) along with paradoxical increase in anal sphincter pressure.

Type I

Type II

Type III

Type IV

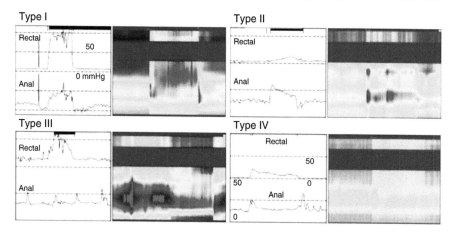

Fig. 5.4 The four types (I–IV) of dyssynergic defecation patterns described in the text are shown using conventional manometry (lines) and HRAM (color topographic plots) (reproduced from Lee et al. [29])

- In type II the patient is unable to generate adequate propulsive forces; additionally there is paradoxical anal contraction.
- In type III the patient can generate adequate propulsive forces, but there is either absent relaxation or inadequate (≤20%) relaxation of anal sphincter.
- In type IV the patient is unable to generate adequate propulsive forces together with an absent or inadequate (≤20%) relaxation of anal sphincter.

Ratuapli et al., by using HRAM in 62 healthy women and 295 women affected by CC, identified three phenotypes (high anal, low rectal, and hybrid) discriminating patients with normal and abnormal balloon expulsion time with 75% sensitivity and 75% specificity, simplifying the previous Rao's classification [30] (Fig. 5.5).

However, several questions exist about the use and the ability of anorectal manometry to diagnose FDD and identify clinical phenotypes: indeed the utility of a negative rectoanal pressure gradient as a marker of FDD is unclear because the gradient values overlap considerably among healthy subjects and constipated patients with and without FDD [33–35].

Another interesting matter of debate is the potential use of HRAM/HDAM in the differential diagnosis between functional and structural abnormalities. A total of 188 consecutive patients with obstructive defecation underwent a full investigation consisting in HRAM and defeco-MR. Compared with patients with dyssynergia on MR imaging, patients with structural pathology, such as rectocele and rectal prolapse, had lower resting and squeeze pressures but a higher rectoanal pressure gradient on HRAM. HRAM diagnostic accuracy for dyssynergia was 82% compared with 77% MR. Interobserver agreement was substantial for HRAM diagnoses. If the data will be confirmed by other studies, these manometric patterns could play a predictive role in identifying patients needing a defecographic study [36].

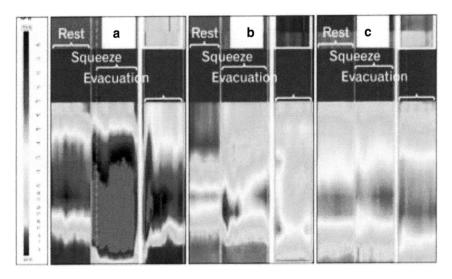

Fig. 5.5 The three defecatory subtypes based on principal components analysis: (**a**) high anal, (**b**) hybrid, and (**c**) low rectal phenotype (reproduced from Ratuapli et al. [30])

5.2.3 Hirschsprung Disease

Hirschsprung disease is characterized by the absence of ganglion cells in the myenteric and submucosal plexus on rectal biopsy.

The absence of the RAIR is known to be a pathognomonic feature of the disease. The absence of RAIR can be explained by the abnormality of the polysynaptic interneurons in the IAS and of the nitrergic inhibitory neurons [37].

The diagnosis is based on the combination of clinical symptoms and results from barium enema, anorectal manometry, and rectal suction biopsy with staining for calretinin or acetylcholinesterase [36–38].

Anorectal manometry has been proved to be a reliable and minimally invasive diagnostic technique: it is a simple screening test in patients with a clinical suspicion of Hirsprung disease. Its most important aim is the differential diagnosis between acquired megacolon and Hirschsprung disease, especially in the ultra-short form of the latter condition.

In infants and children, an absent RAIR has a sensitivity of 91% and a specificity of 94% for the diagnosis of Hirschsprung disease [39]. These figures are slightly but not significantly lower than rectal suction biopsy. When RAIR is present, it excludes an Hirschsprung disease diagnosis.

HRAM is an effective and safe method for the diagnosis in newborns as demonstrated by Tang, who reported a sensitivity of 89% and a specificity of 83% [40].

Wu et al. performed ARM in a group of 24 infants (eight with Hirschsprung disease and 16 without) and HRAM in a group of 21 infants (nine with Hirschsprung disease and 12 without). The authors assessed RAIR adequacy by calculating the sphincter relaxation integral (ASRI) during the HRAM study at pressure cutoff <10, <15, and <20 mmHg (ASRI10, ASRI15, and ASRI20) and investigated their diagnostic utility. They concluded that ASRI10 may be an indicative cutoff for the adequacy of RAIR in infants [41].

Many children with Hirschsprung disease have good surgical results; however, unfortunately, some patients continue to have persistent bowel dysfunction such as constipation and intestinal motility disturbance. The postoperative anorectal manometric evaluation of the patients after surgery provides detailed information about the function of anal canal and rectum. Demirbag et al. evaluated with ARM 18 children after surgery and found an absent RAIR in 14 (77.7%) and an abnormal RAIR in 4 (22.2%). They concluded that the majority of the patients have impaired anorectal motility after surgery but the manometric evaluation did not provide enough information in understanding the causes of symptoms. It is hoped that the new HRAM/HDAM techniques will help to solve this important issue [9].

5.2.4 Pelvic Floor Rehabilitation

Pelvic floor retraining is frequently recommended for defecation disorders. However, the lack of patient's selections and the lack of homogeneity of rehabilitation methods and protocols jeopardize the results causing difficulty in evaluation outcomes [42].

Jodorkovsky et al. retrospectively reviewed 203 patients, who had previously undergone HRAM, in whom manometric results were used for recommending biofeedback as treatment strategy. Biofeedback was ultimately recommended in 119 (58%) patients (80 with CC, 27 with FI, 9 with a combination of CC and FI, and 3 with rectal pain), of whom only 51 actually received therapy. 38 out of 51 underwent at least five sessions of biofeedback, with real life outcome success reported in 66% [43].

Soubra et al. performed HRAM on 25 patients awaiting biofeedback for dyssynergic defecation previously diagnosed through ARM. HRAM pressures tended to be higher than conventional ARM. Although there was high consensus regarding diagnosis of dyssynergia, there was low correlation regarding pattern types. For these reasons, the authors concluded that new diagnostic pressure criteria should be adopted in centers converting to HRAM [44].

5.3   HRAM/HDAM: Potentialities and Perspectives

HRAM and HDAM offer the possibility to have a standardized technique for performing the exam. Moreover, new parameters have been recently studied and developed both in HRAM and HDAM and are being considered for a future introduction in clinical practice.

Without any doubt, the most important gain over conventional ARM is the better capability in studying and understanding the functional anatomy of the sphincter since the distribution of the pressures in the anal canal and the possible asymmetry on the axial and on the circumferential plane are clearly shown [45].

Rezaie et al. studied 39 patients using both endoanal ultrasound (EUS), which is the gold standard for detecting anal sphincter defect, and HDAM. As there was no standard protocol for classifying a sphincter defect using HDAM, they defined sphincter defect as any pressure measurement below 25 mmHg with the canal anal at rest, involving at least 18° of the whole anal circumference (Fig. 5.6) [46].

The authors achieved a sensitivity, specificity, and NPV of 74%, 75%, and 92%, respectively, but a PPV of only 43%. The notable NPV of 92% is promising suggesting that HDAM may be useful in ruling out a sphincter defect helping to better select patients to suggest also EUS.

HRAM could be also used to provide a new classification of FDD as shown by Ratuapli et al. who studied 62 healthy females and 295 females with FDD. They demonstrated that three phenotypes, characterized by (1) high anal pressure at rest and during evacuation ("high anal"), (2) low rectal pressure alone ("low rectal"), and (3) low rectal pressure with impaired anal relaxation during evacuation ("hybrid") were able to discriminate between patients with normal and abnormal prolonged balloon expulsion time (BET) [30].

HDAM could shed new light also on the paradoxical contraction of puborectalis muscle as demonstrated by Xu et al. [47] who evaluated 71 healthy adults and 79 patients with paradoxical puborectalis syndrome (PPS). They found that the pressures were high in the proximal circumferential wall of anorectum in healthy adults and, in contrast, the pressures were low in the proximal circumferential wall of anorectum during simulated defecation in patients with PPS. A characteristic high-pressure area ("boot shaped"), highlighted in the distal posterior wall of the anorectum, was absent in healthy adults.

So, differently from ARM, HDAM could be as important as defecography and electromyography in the diagnosis of PPS.

Moreover HDAM is able to provide additional information about structure and function of the anorectum, which would be unavailable with 2D analysis alone, as shown by Raja et al. who found that the puborectalis tone was absent at rest more often in patients with FI than in those with constipation. Besides, the analysis of 3D images also provided the identification of 29 focal defects not seen with 2D analysis. Furthermore, 3D image analysis allowed the identification of 29 focal defects that had not previously been detected with 2D image analysis [14].

Some new HRAM and HDAM parameters have been recently described and could be used in differentiating patients with dyssynergic defecation and healthy subjects: the anal contractile integral (ACI), the post contraction pressure (PSP), the integrated pressure of the anal relaxation (aIRP), and the sliding speed of the probe during the squeeze in the anal canal (SVAC). In a study involving 40 healthy volunteers (28 women, median age 35 years) and 20 patients with dyssynergic defecation (12 women, median age 46 years), the patients with dyssynergic defecation showed significant different values in comparison with healthy volunteers for each of the

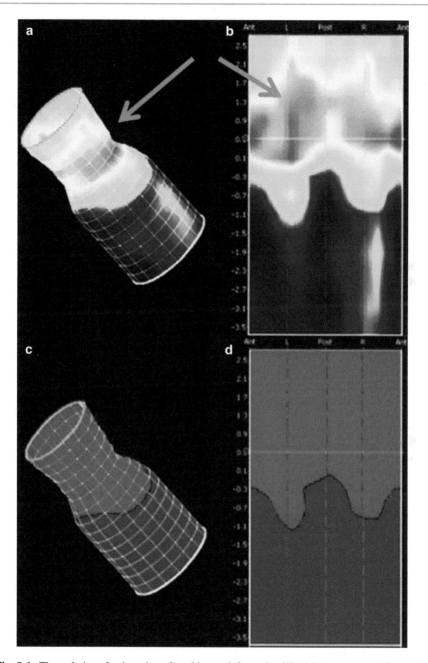

Fig. 5.6 The technique for detection of a sphincter defect using HDAM. An anterior defect while recording resting pressure is shown in (**a**, **b**). The defect becomes more visible when minimum and maximum ranges are set at 24 and 25 mmHg (orange arrows) (**c**, **d**). Using this technique, the extent of the defect was calculated to be 149° by dividing the length of orange arrows by the circumference of the anal canal (reproduced from Rezaie et al. [46])

parameters above described. Up to now, it is too early to state if these parameters will be able to clearly distinguish normal subjects from patients and further studies are mandatory for their validation [48].

Pandolfino et al. in 2008 proposed a novel concept of integrated pressurized volume (IPV), which is calculated by multiplying amplitude, distance, and a certain time period. This new parameter, after further validation studies, could be also used to provide a precise measurement of muscular contractility of the anal canal [49].

Seo et al. identified five regions separated by a distance of 1 cm from the rectum (6 cm from the distal tip of the catheter) to the anus (1 cm from the distal tip of the catheter) (Fig. 5.7). The IPV of each portion and the IPV ratio, which were obtained with and without balloon distention, were compared to determine the value that most precisely predicted the results of the balloon expulsion test. They showed that the ratio of the integrated pressurized volume of the upper 1-cm portion to those of the lower 4-cm portion (IPV14 ratio) with balloon distention was better at predicting balloon expulsion time. They concluded that these novel manometric parameter could be more effective in predicting balloon expulsion time than conventional parameters based on linear waves at certain signal points along the anal canal [50].

Moreover, HRAM and especially HDAM could be useful in the diagnosis of structural anorectal disorders, like the perineum descending syndrome and rectal intussusception, even if further observations on larger samples are needed [46].

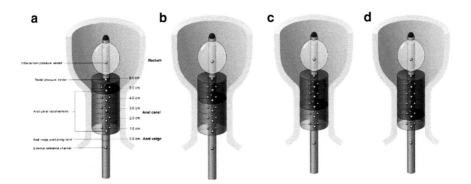

Fig. 5.7 Four categories of integrated pressurized volume (IPV) from the rectum to the anal canal (**a–d**). (**a**) The pressure signals obtained during simulated evacuation from the rectum (6 cm from the distal tip of the catheter) to the upper margin of the anal canal (5 cm from the distal tip of the catheter) were considered to belong to the upper 1-cm portion of the anorectal canal (red), whereas those from the upper margin of the anal canal (5 cm from the distal tip of the catheter) to the distal margin of the anal canal (1 cm from distal tip of the catheter) were considered to belong to the lower 4-cm portion of the anorectal canal (blue). The ratio of the upper 1-cm portion to the lower 4-cm portion can be considered as the ratio of the volume of the red-colored portion to that of the blue-colored portion. (**b**) IPVs from the upper 2-cm portion (red) and IPVs from the lower 3-cm portion (blue) (**c**) IPVs from the upper 3-cm portion (red) and IPVs from the lower 2-cm portion (blue) (**d**) IPVs from the upper 4-cm portion (red) and IPVs from the lower 1-cm portion (blue) (reproduced from Seo et al. [50])

Vitton et al., using HDAM in a patient with long history of intractable constipation, found an incomplete anal relaxation during attempted defecation, indicating a pelvic floor dyssynergia and a 9 mm perineal descent on the manometric probe. At the end of the bear down the perineum gained its initial position indicating that the probe had not moved [51]. In this patient also the conventional defecography showed a 9.2 mm perineal descent from the puborectalis line. This first observation was then confirmed by Benezech et al. in 19 female patients with excessive perineal descent diagnosed by defecography. They concluded that HDAM can diagnose excessive perineal descent with the same degree of reliability as defecography [52] (Fig. 5.8).

Also Heinrich et al. supported the hypothesis that HRAM might help to distinguish defecatory disorders due to functional or structural causes. In their study, an elevated intrarectal pressure above a narrow band of high pressure in the anal canal seemed to be associated with rectal intussusceptions [53].

Benezech et al. [54] using HDAM in 26 patients presented with rectal intussusceptions showed that 21 of them had an elevated intrarectal pressure above a narrow band of high pressure in the anal canal during straining, defined as a rectal intussusception as previously described by Heinrich [53]. This additional high-pressure area was located at the superior anterior edge of the probe in 13 patients, at the superior posterior edge in six patients, and at the superior anterior and posterior edge in two patients. (Fig. 5.9). Using these data, the most relevant diagnostic

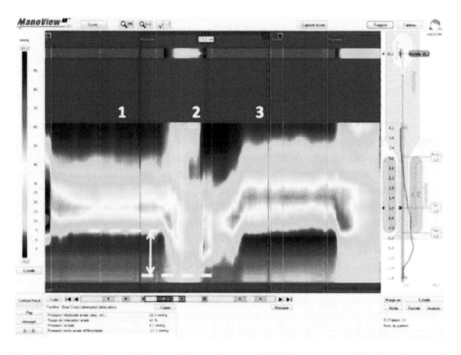

Fig. 5.8 Perineal descent: the row between the two dotted line measures the size of perineal descent (reproduced from Benezech et al. [52])

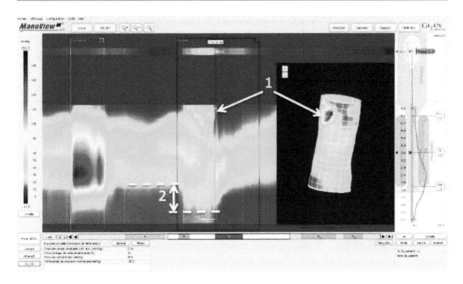

Fig. 5.9 (1) Rectal intussusception is an elevated intrarectal pressure above a narrow band of high pressure in the anal canal during straining; (2) excessive perineal descent (reproduced from Benezech et al. [54])

criterion with the best Yuden Index (0.69) was the association between an anterior additional high-pressure area and a perineal descent, with a positive predictive value of 100%, a negative predictive value of 61.9%, a specificity of 100%, and a sensitivity of 69.2%.

However, up to now, defecography remains the gold standard for the diagnosis of rectal intussusception and the results with HDAM must be compared and integrated with those obtained using conventional X-ray defecography and/or MR defecography [55, 56].

Also Prichard et al. [57] compared HRAM and MR defecography in healthy subjects and in patients with rectal prolapse. Among patients with rectal prolapse, there were two phenotypes, which were characterized by high (PC1) or lower (PC2) anal pressure at rest and squeeze along with higher rectal and anal pressure (PC1) or a higher rectoanal gradient during evacuation (PC2). PC1 and PC2 explained 48% and 31% of the variance, respectively. PC1 was correlated with higher anal pressures at rest and squeeze and higher rectal and anal pressures during evacuation. In contrast, PC2 was inversely correlated with anal pressures at rest and during squeeze; PC2 was correlated with a greater rectoanal pressure gradient during evacuation. In a logistic model, the PC1 score adjusted for age discriminated between controls and rectal prolapse with accuracy of 96%.

Brusciano et al. [58] investigated the correlation between rectal wall thickness (RWT) and rectal pressure (RP), using 3D endorectal ultrasound (3D-EUS) and HRAM, in patients with obstructed defecation syndrome (ODS) caused by internal rectal prolapse. They measured four rectal segments thickness (RWTs) introducing a new parameter, as the total rectal wall volume (TRWV). They found that in ODS patients there was a significant lower TRWV than in healthy volunteers (62.8% with mild and 28% with severe impairment). They also found, as previously reported in other studies that a lower rectoanal gradient was related with constipation symptoms [59, 60].

5.4 Conclusions

In conclusion, HRAM and HDAM are more intuitive and relatively simpler to perform than the ARM. They are very promising for improving the evaluation of functional alterations of the anal canal and the pelvic floor; indeed, they improve the understanding of the anorectal pathophysiology, allowing more precise correlation between anatomy and function. e.g. better evaluating the spontaneous activity of the anal canal, sometimes difficult to assess with the conventional technique.

The standardization of the new HRAM/HDAM parameters, which could add a further diagnostic yield in the study of motor and functional anorectal disorders, will probably require longer time periods. It will be mandatory to study large well-selected groups of patients and healthy subjects different for age, gender, parity and, probably, ethnicity.

References

1. Scott SM, Gladman MA. Manometric, sensorimotor, and neurophysiologic evaluation of anorectal function. Gastroenterol Clin N Am. 2008;37(3):511–38.
2. Carrington EV, Scott SM, Bharucha A, Mion F, Remes-Troche JM, Malcolm A, et al. Expert consensus document: advances in the evaluation of anorectal function. Nat Rev Gastroenterol Hepatol. 2018;15(5):309–23.
3. Lam TJ, Felt-Bersma RJ. Women with chronic constipation: clinical examination is more important than anorectal function testing. Ned Tijdschr Geneeskd. 2013;157(8):A5665.
4. Hallan RI, Marzouk D, Waldron DJ, Womack NR, Williams NS. Comparison of digital and manometric assessment of anal sphincter function. Br J Surg. 1989;76:973–5.
5. Diamant NE, Kamm MA, Wald A, Whitehead WE. AGA technical review on anorectal testing techniques. Gastroenterology. 1999;116(3):735–60.
6. Heinrich H, Fruehauf H, Sauter M, Steingötter A, Fried M, Schwizer W, et al. The effect of standard compared to enhanced instruction and verbal feedback on anorectal manometry measurements. Neurogastroenterol Motil. 2013;25(3):230–7.
7. Basilisco G, Bharucha AE. High-resolution anorectal manometry: An expensive hobby or worth every penny? Neurogastroenterol Motil. 2017;29(8):13125.
8. Grossi U, Carrington EV, Bharucha AE, Horrocks EJ, Scott SM, Knowles CH. Diagnostic accuracy study of anorectal manometry for diagnosis of dyssynergic defecation. Gut. 2016;65(3):447–55.
9. Demirbag S, Tiryaki T, Purtuloglu T. Importance of anorectal manometry after definitive surgery for Hirschsprung's disease in children. Afr J Paediatr Surg. 2013;10(1):1–4.
10. Bajwa A, Thiruppathy K, Emmanuel A. The utility of conditioning sequences in barostat protocols for the measurements of rectal compliance. Color Dis. 2013;15(6):715–8.
11. Jones MP, Post J, Crowell MD. High-resolution manometry in the evaluation of anorectal disorders: a simultaneous comparison with water-perfused manometry. Am J Gastroenterol. 2007;102(4):850–5.

12. Ambartsumyan L, Rodriguez L, Morera C, Nurko S. Longitudinal and radial characteristics of intra-anal pressures in children using 3D high-definition anorectal manometry: new observations. Am J Gastroenterol. 2013;108(12):1918–28.
13. Kang HR, Lee JE, Lee JS, Lee TH, Hong SJ, Kim JO, et al. Comparison of high-resolution anorectal manometry with water-perfused anorectal manometry. J Neurogastroenterol Motil. 2015;21(1):126–32.
14. Raja S, Okeke FC, Stein EM, Dhalla S, Nandwani M, Lynch KL, Gyawali CP, Clarke JO. Three-dimensional anorectal manometry enhances diagnostic gain by detecting sphincter defects and puborectalis pressure. Dig Dis Sci. 2017;62(12):3536–41.
15. Damon H, Guye O, Seigneurin A, et al. Prevalence of anal incontinence in adults and impact on quality of life. Gastroenterol Clin Biol. 2006;30:37–43.
16. Bharucha AE, Dunivan G, Goode PS, et al. Epidemiology, pathophysiology, and classification of fecal incontinence: state of the science summary for the National Institute of Diabetes and Digestive and Kidney Diseases (NIDDK) workshop. Am J Gastroenterol. 2015;110:127–36.
17. Bharucha AE, Rao SS. An update on anorectal disorders for gastroenterologists. Gastroenterology. 2014;146(1):37–45.e2.
18. Mion F, Garros A, Brochard C, Vitton V, Ropert A, Bouvier M, et al. 3D high-definition anorectal manometry : values obtained in asymptomatic volunteers, fecal incontinence and chronic constipation. Results of a prospective multicenter study (NOMAD). Neurogastroenterol Motil. 2017;29(8):13049.
19. Bharucha AE, Fletcher JG, Harper CM, et al. Relationship between symptoms and disordered continence mechanisms in women with idiopathic faecal incontinence. Gut. 2005;54:546–55.
20. Whitehead WE, Borrud L, Goode PS, et al. Fecal incontinence in US adults: epidemiology and risk factors. Gastroenterology. 2009;137(2):512–7.
21. McHugh SM, Diamant NE. Anal canal pressure profile: a reappraisal as determined by rapid pullthrough technique. Gut. 1987;28:1234–41.
22. Raizada V, Bhargava V, Karsten A, et al. Functional morphology of anal sphincter complex unveiled by high definition anal manometery and three dimensional ultrasound imaging. Neurogastroenterol Motil. 2011;23(11):1013–9.
23. Carrington EV, Knowles CH, Grossi U, Scott SM. High-resolution anorectal manometry measures are more accurate than conventional measures in detecting anal hypocontractility in women with fecal incontinence. Clin Gastroenterol Hepatol. 2019;17(3):477–485.e9.
24. Higgins PD, Johanson JF. Epidemiology of constipation in North America: a systematic review. Am J Gastroenterol. 2004;99(4):750–9.
25. Bellini M, Gambaccini D, Salvadori S, Bocchini R, Pucciani F, Bove A, Alduini P, Battaglia E, Bassotti G. Different perception of chronic constipation between patients and gastroenterologists. Neurogastroenterol Motil. 2018;30:e13336.
26. Bharucha AE, Dorn SD, Lembo A, Pressman A, American Gastroenterological Association. American gastroenterological association medical position statement on constipation. Gastroenterology. 2013;144(1):211–7.
27. Rao SS, Bharucha AE, Chiarioni G, Felt-Bersma R, Knowles C, Malcolm A, et al. Functional anorectal disorders. Gastroenterology. 2016;150:1430–42.
28. Rao SSC, Tuteja AK, Vellema T, et al. Dyssynergic defecation: demographics, symptoms, stool patterns, and quality of life. J Clin Gastroenterol. 2004;38:680–5.
29. Lee YY, Erdogan A, Yu S, Dewitt A, Rao SSC. Anorectal manometry in defecatory disorders: a comparative analysis of high-resolution pressure topography and waveform manometry. J Neurogastroenterol Motil. 2018;24(3):460–8.
30. Ratuapli S, Bharucha AE, Noelting J, et al. Phenotypic identification and classification of functional defecatory disorders using high resolution anorectal manometry. Gastroenterology. 2013;144:314–22.
31. Duthie GS, Bartolo DC. Anismus: the cause of constipation? Results of investigation and treatment. World J Surg. 1992;16(5):831–5.

32. Dinning PG, Bampton PA, Andre J, Kennedy ML, Lubowski DZ, King DW, et al. Abnormal predefecatory colonic motor patterns define constipation in obstructed defecation. Gastroenterology. 2004;127(1):49–56.
33. Rao SS, Welcher KD, Leistikow JS. Obstructive defecation: a failure of rectoanal coordination. Am J Gastroenterol. 1998;93:1042–50.
34. Ratuapli S, Bharucha AE, Harvey D, et al. Comparison of rectal balloon expulsion test in seated and left lateral positions. Neurogastroenterol Motil. 2013;25(12):e813–20.
35. Rao SS, Mudipalli RS, Stessman M, et al. Investigation of the utility of colorectal function tests and Rome II criteria in dyssynergic defecation (anismus). Neurogastroenterol Motil. 2004;16:589–96.
36. Heinrich H, Sauter M, Fox M, Weishaupt D, Halama M, Misselwitz B, et al. Assessment of obstructive defecation by high-resolution anorectal manometry compared with magnetic resonance defecography. Clin Gastroenterol Hepatol. 2015;13(7):1310–7.
37. Matsufuji H, Yokoyama J. Neural control of the internal anal sphincter motility. J Smooth Muscle Res. 2003;39(1–2):11–20.
38. Musa ZA, Qasim BJ, Ghazi HF, Al Shaikhly AW. Diagnostic roles of calretinin in Hirschsprung disease: a comparison to neuron-specific enolase. Saudi J Gastroenterol. 2017;23:60–6.
39. De Lorijn F, Kremer LC, Reitsma JB, Benninga MA. Diagnostic tests in Hirschsprung disease: a systematic review. J Pediatr Gastroenterol Nutr. 2006;42(5):496–505.
40. Tang YF, Chen JG, An HJ, Jin P, Yang L, Dai ZF, et al. High-resolution anorectal manometry in newborns: normative values and diagnostic utility in Hirschsprung disease. Neurogastroenterol Motil. 2014;26:1565–72.
41. Wu JF, Lu CH, Yang CH, Tsai IJ. Diagnostic role of anal sphincter relaxation integral in high-resolution anorectal manometry for Hirschsprung disease in infants. J Pediatr. 2018;194:136–141.e2.
42. Bocchini R, Chiarioni G, Corazziari E, Pucciani F, Torresan F, Alduini P, Bassotti G, Battaglia E, Ferrarini F, Galeazzi F, Londoni C, Rossitti P, Usai Satta P, Iona L, Marchi S, Milazzo G, Altomare DF, Barbera R, Bove A, Calcara C, D'Alba L, De Bona M, Goffredo F, Manfredi G, Naldini G, Neri MC, Turco L, La Torre F, D'Urso AP, Berni I, Balestri MA, Busin N, Boemo C, Bellini M. Pelvic floor rehabilitation for defecation disorders. Tech Coloproctol. 2019;23(2):101–15.
43. Jodorkovsky D, Macura KJ, Gearhart SL, Dunbar KB, Stein EM, Clarke JO. High-resolution anorectal manometry and dynamic pelvic magnetic resonance imaging are complementary technologies. J Gastroenterol Hepatol. 2015;30(1):71–4.
44. Soubra M, Go J, Valestin J, Schey RA. Comparison of standard anorectal manometry and high resolution manometry pattern in dyssynergic patients. J Gastroenterol Hepatol Res. 2014;3:1244–7.
45. Raizada V, Bhargava V, Karsten A, et al. Functional morphology of anal sphincter complex unveiled by high definition anal manometry and three-dimensional ultrasound imaging. Neurogastroenterol Motil. 2011;23(11):1013–9.
46. Rezaie A, Iriana S, Pimentel M, et al. Can three-dimensional high-resolution anorectal manometry detect anal sphincter defects in patients with faecal incontinence? Color Dis. 2016;19(5):468–75.
47. Xu C, Zhao R, Conklin JL, et al. Three-dimensional high-resolution anorectal manometry in the diagnosis of paradoxical puborectalis syndrome compared with healthy adults: a retrospective study in 79 cases. Eur J Gastroenterol Hepatol. 2014;26(6):621–9.
48. Remes-Troche JM, Roesch FB, Azamar-Jacome A. topography and characterization of anal ultraslow waves (AUSWs) in patients with proctalgia fugax. A study using high-definition anorectal manometry (HDM). Gastroenterology. 2012;143(5 Suppl 1):905.
49. Pandolfino JE, Ghosh SK, Rice J, Clarke JO, Kwaiatek MA, Hahrilas PJ. Classifying esophageal motility by pressure topography characteristics: a study of 400 patients and 75 controls. Am J Gastroenterol. 2008;103:1510–8.

50. Seo M, Joo S, Jung KW, et al. A high-resolution anorectal manometry parameter based on integrated pressurized volume: a study based on 204 male patients with constipation and 26 controls. Neurogastroenterol Motil. 2018;30(9):e13376.
51. Vitton V, Grimaud JC, Bouvier M. Three-dimension high-resolution anorectal manometry can precisely measure perineal descent. J Neurogastroenterol Motil. 2013;19(2):257–8.
52. Benezech A, Bouvier M, Grimaud JC, Baumstarck K, Vitton V. Three-dimensional high-resolution anorectal manometry and diagnosis of excessive perineal descent: a comparative pilot study with defaecography. Color Dis. 2014;16(5):O170–5.
53. Heinrich H, Sauter M, Fox M, Weishaupt D, Halama M, Misselwitz B, Buetikofer S, Reiner C, Fried M, Schwizer W, Fruehauf H. Assessment of obstructive defecation by high-resolution anorectal manometry compared with magnetic resonance defecography. Clin Gastroenterol Hepatol. 2015;13(7):1310–7.
54. Benezech A, Cappiello M, Baumstarck K, Grimaud JC, Bouvier M, Vitton V. Rectal intussusception: can high resolution three-dimensional ano-rectal manometry compete with conventional defecography? Neurogastroenterol Motil. 2017;29(4):12978.
55. Remes Troche JM, Pérez Luna E, Reyes Huerta JU, et al. Development of new parameters to evaluate anorectal function using high-definition anorectal manometry (HDM). The anal contractile integrated (ACI), the post squeeze pressure (PSP), the anal integrated relaxation pressure (aIRP), and the sliding velocity in the anal canal (SVAC). Gastroenterology. 2013;144(5):S365.
56. Jung KW, Joo S, Yang DH, et al. A novel high-resolution anorectal manometry parameter based on a three-dimensional integrated pressurized volume of a spatiotemporal plot, for predicting balloon expulsion in asymptomatic normal individuals. Neurogastroenterol Motil. 2014;26(7):937–49.
57. Prichard DO, Lee T, Parthasarathy G, Fletcher JG, Zinsmeister AR, Bharucha AE. High-resolution anorectal manometry for identifying defecatory disorders and rectal structural abnormalities in women. Clin Gastroenterol Hepatol. 2017;15(3):412–20.
58. Brusciano L, Tolone S, Limongelli P, Del Genio G, Messina F, Martellucci J, Volpe ML, Longo A, Docimo L. Anatomical and functional features of the internal rectal prolapse with outlet obstruction determined with 3D endorectal ultrasonography and high-resolution anorectal manometry: an observational case-control study. Am J Gastroenterol. 2018;113(8):1247–50.
59. Zani A, Eaton S, Morini F, Puri P, Rintala R, Heurn EV, et al. European Paediatric Surgeons' Association survey on the management of Hirschsprung disease. Eur J Pediatr Surg. 2017;27:96–101.
60. Noelting J, Ratuapli SK, Bharucha AE, Harvey DM, Ravi K, Zinsmeister AR. Normal values for high-resolution anorectal manometry in healthy women: effects of age and significance of rectoanal gradient. Am J Gastroenterol. 2012;107(10):1530–6.

Technical Aspects and Equipment

6

Claudio Londoni, Salvatore Tolone, Andrea Pancetti, and Lorenzo Bertani

During anorectal manometry, the evaluation of anal and rectal pressure is carried out using an intra-rectal catheter connected, through pressure transducers, to an acquisition system. A dedicated software elaborates the data showing the recorded pressures and allowing automatic and manual analysis [1–3].

While older, "non-high resolution" catheters have from three to eight unidirectional sensors, high resolution anorectal manometry (HRAM) and high definition anorectal manometry (HDAM) catheters contain several closely spaced circumferential sensor elements along the longitudinal axis. The pressure-sensing element varies among systems.

1. In catheters manufactured by Given Imaging, a Medtronic Company (Yoqneam, Israel), this comprises 256 pressure sensors (ManoScan HD-AM catheter) or 12 channels: each channel consists in 12 radial pressure sensors, 144 electronic sensors in total (ManoScan HR-AM catheter).
2. Unisensor catheters (UniTip, Attikon, Switzerland) are comprised of a unidirectional pressure sensor embedded within a soft membrane containing silicone gel [4].
3. The catheter manufactured by Sandhill has 4 radially arranged sensors at each level [5].
4. Water-perfused high resolution catheters (Mui Scientific, Mississauga, Ontario, Canada) are also available.

C. Londoni (✉)
Gastroenterology and Digestive Endoscopy Unit, ASST-Maggiore Hospital, Crema, Italy

S. Tolone
General, Mininvasive and Obesity Surgery Unit, Departement of Advanced Medical and Surgical Sciences, University of Campania "Luigi Vanvitelli", Naples, Italy

A. Pancetti · L. Bertani
Department of New Technologies and Translational Research in Medicine and Surgery, Gastroenterology Unit, University of Pisa, Pisa, Italy

© Springer Nature Switzerland AG 2020
M. Bellini (ed.), *High Resolution and High Definition Anorectal Manometry*,
https://doi.org/10.1007/978-3-030-32419-3_6

Table 6.1 Qualitative comparison of HRAM and HDAM catheters versus non-high resolution anorectal manometry catheters

	HRAM and HDAM	Non-HRM
Number of sensors	Closely spaced more sensors	Fewer sensors at wider intervals
Display	Color contour and line plot	Line plot
Techniques	Stationary examination	Pull-through examination
Preparation	Easy	More time consuming
Spatiotemporal resolution	Good	Limited
Cost	High	Low
Catheter durability	Limited	Excellent
Lifespan	Limited	Excellent

HRAM and non-HRAM catheters are compared in Table 6.1. HRAM and HDAM catheters provide a continuous and dynamic spatiotemporal mapping of anorectal pressures, allowing easier and more detailed data interpretation [6, 7].

6.1   Conventional Anorectal Manometry

Water-perfused manometry requires more preparation, technical skills, and training [4]. The dynamic performance of water-perfused systems is several orders of magnitude less than that of solid-state systems, limiting their accuracy where rapidly changing pressures must be measured (e.g., in the pharynx/upper esophageal sphincter) [4]. However, this is not a limitation in the anorectum where rapidly changing pressures are not observed.

The conventional anorectal manometry water-perfused system consists of (Fig.6.1) the following:

1. Polygraph.
2. Dedicated software.
3. Water perfusion pump.
4. Single-use or multipurpose water-perfused catheter with four or eight channels.
5. Pressure transducers.

The catheter capillaries are filled with water and constantly perfused through the pump (0.5–1 mL/min); it is necessary to do a periodical check of the perfusion flow counting the numbers of the water drops per minute (20 drops = 1 mL). At the exit of each capillary a constant quantity of water flows at a constant speed. The capillaries are connected to the pressure transducers and these are connected to the polygraph [2, 3].

The pressure exerted at the exit point of the capillaries is transmitted to the whole water column inside the capillary and is transformed into an electrical signal by the pressure transducer. The electrical signal is transmitted to the polygraph which, through the software, represents it on the computer screen. The pressure

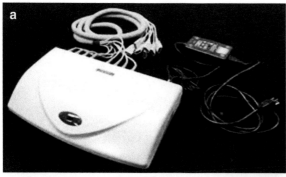

MEDTRONIC

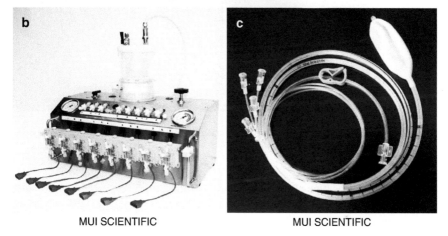

MUI SCIENTIFIC   MUI SCIENTIFIC

Fig. 6.1 (**a**) Polygraph dedicated software, (**b**) Water perfusion pump, (**c**) Single-use or multipurpose water-perfused catheter with four channels

measurement performed through the catheter is carried out at a constant frequency, so that the resulting graphic representation is a wave with time on the X axis and pressure values on the Y axis (Fig. 6.2) [2, 3].

The catheter configuration can be different regarding the number of channels (four, six, or eight) and their spatial arrangement which can be as follows:

1. Fully radial.
2. Fully helicoidal.
3. Mix between the two previous provisions.

A disposable catheter of a latex free material is generally used.

Although the procedure does not present any particular difficulties, it is important to take into account some technical aspects that could affect the quality of the manometric exam:

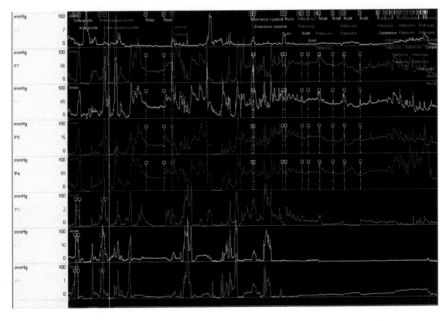

Fig. 6.2 The graphic representation of conventional anorectal manometry. Time on the X axis and pressure values on the Y axis (Laborie-Software)

- Regardless of the type of the configuration of the catheter, the pressure measurements take place in a unidirectional manner: the pressure is evaluated only at the point where the water exits out of the capillary; no information about the pressure from other areas is available.
- The water perfusion, produced by the pneumatic pump, has to be constant and equal for all the channels.
- It is mandatory to calibrate the catheter at two different levels holding the horizontal catheter at the level of the couch before, low level, and then at high level, 50 cm above low level.
- To avoid false pressure values, it is extremely important to maintain the catheter at the same level during all procedure (low calibration level: 0 mmHg).
- During the different phases of the manometric test, it is necessary to move the catheter inside the anal canal manually or by using a mechanical extractor controlled by the software.

6.2 High-Resolution Water-Perfused Manometry (HRWPM)

The way HRAM perfused system works is similar to the conventional system seen above, except for the increased number of catheter channels (up to 24) [1, 8, 9].

Obviously the polygraph and the software have to be able to manage this increased number of channels and, hence, this increased amount of information.

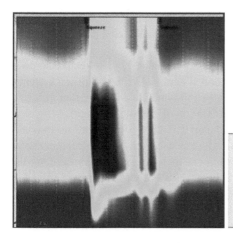
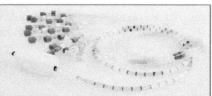

Fig. 6.3 The graphic representation of high resolution water-perfused manometry. The contour plot with isobaric colored representation. On the right side of the figure, there is a catheter with increased number of channels (Laborie-MMS origin)

The catheter, made of bio-compatible plastic material, can be single-use or multipurpose (50 uses are generally permitted after autoclaving).

The increased number of channels provides a greater detail of the rectal and anal pressures allowing to obtain a more accurate examination.

One critical point is maintaining a constant perfusion of all the channels. This is even more necessary than conventional ARM and before starting the examination the operator has often to spend some time to perform the setup (e.g., to verify that all transducers are correctly connected and all channels are really working). Also HRWPM requires that the catheter and the acquisition system are placed at the same level.

In comparison with conventional water-perfused ARM the increased number of channels allows to maintain the catheter in place during the examination without needing to change its position. This aspect speeds up the execution of the exam itself.

The software can display pressures via linear track and as contour plot (Fig. 6.3). This last type of visualization is typical of high resolution manometric examinations and allows to have a continuous representation of pressure through an isobaric colored representation of immediate comprehension [1, 8, 9].

6.3   Solid-State High Resolution Manometry

The high resolution anorectal manometry system using solid-state catheter requires the following:

1. Acquisition module.
2. Dedicated software.
3. Solid-state multi-use catheter (electronic pressure transducers).
4. Single-use balloons.

In this case, the pressure transducers are integrated into the catheter; they are electronic sensors that modify the intensity of the electrical signal proportionally to the pressure variations.

The pressures recorded with this method are not influenced by the reciprocal position between the transducers and the acquisition system, unlike the perfusion systems.

There are several solid-state anorectal catheters available on the market differing in number of channels, and number and orientation of pressure sensors.

For the Given Imaging, a Medtronic Company HRAM-system, there are two versions of this solid-state catheter (ManoScan AR catheter), which has an outer diameter of 4.2 mm. The regular probe (AAN) has ten channels at 6-mm intervals along the anal canal and two channels in the rectal balloon: 12 electronic sensors are placed in each channel (Fig. 6.4a). The small probe (APN) has seven channels along the anal canal and more one channel in the rectal balloon: 12 electronic sensors are placed in each channel. The manufacturer recommends a latex free rectal balloon that is 3.3 cm long and has a maximal capacity of 400 mL. Indeed the manufacturer's recommended rectal balloons for all HRAM catheters cited in this review have similar dimensions.

For the Sandhill HRAM system the probe of the solid-state system (4-mm outer diameter; Sandhill Scientific, Denver, CO, USA) has eight directional sensors. The most proximal sensor is placed in the rectal balloon (latex-free; maximal capacity 400 ml). Distally to that there is a rectum sensor, and then five anal sensors, each separated by 10 mm; an external reference pressure sensor is located 1 cm outside the anal verge (Fig. 6.4b). The sphincter pressure is the average of the pressures recorded by the anal sensors [6].

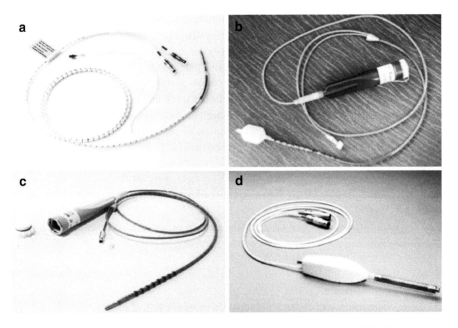

Fig. 6.4 (**a**) Given Imaging, a Medtronic Company HRAM-catheter; (**b**) Sandhill HRAM catheter; (**c**) Unisensor HRAM catheter; (**d**) Solid-state multi-use HD 3D catheter

The Unisensor HRAM system has a 12 Fr probe (4 mm; UniTip, UniSensor, Switzerland) (Fig. 6.4c) with eight pressure sensors. Six sensors, each equidistant from each other, span 5 cm. Then there is a sensor, located 2.5 cm, proximally to the other ones, inside a non-latex balloon with a maximum capacity of 400 mL and a distal sensor, located 2 cm beyond the last anal sensor, which acts as an external reference [10].

According to the different types of catheters on the market, it is possible to have up to 144 pressure sensors arranged radially for a precise and detailed pressure measurement.

The whole area of high pressure generated by the anal sphincters is visualized through a contour plot representation. The sphincter pressure profile is always visible in every phase of the procedure: at rest, during squeezing and straining, and when balloon is progressively filled with increasing air volumes.

It is not necessary to move the catheter during the procedure: the sphincter movements are "monitored" during the analysis by modifying, if necessary, the measurement markers on the screen during data acquisition.

The eSleeve option in the software reduces pressures recorded across the longitudinal extent of the anal canal into a single value. At rest, during squeezing and rectal distention the eSleeve identifies the highest of all pressures recorded by anal sensors at every point in time. This eSleeve value is used to calculate the average and maximum anal resting pressure and the maximum squeeze pressure over 20 seconds during these maneuvers [10].

6.4　High Definition 3D Solid-State Manometry (HDAM)

The HDAM requires the following:

1. Acquisition module.
2. Dedicated software.
3. Solid-state multi-use catheter (electronic pressure transducers) (Fig. 6.4d).
4. Single-use sheath with an end tip balloon.

HDAM probe has 256 circumferentially oriented pressure-sensing elements arranged in 16 rows. Each sensor is spaced from the other 4 mm axially and 2 mm radially. The probe is 6.4 cm in length with a diameter of 10.75 mm. A disposable sheath is necessary (Fig. 6.5): it has a balloon at its tip made of non-latex thermoplastic with a maximum capacity of 400 mL. The balloon has to be fixed to the probe by a Luer-lock connection. The probe is larger and stiffer than other HRAM probes but it is only able to display pressures recorded by individual sensors around the circumference [10]. On the catheter handpiece there is a marker necessary to correctly place (on the posterior wall of the anal canal) the probe inside the rectum.

It is mandatory to calibrate the probe in a calibration chamber where it is zeroed to atmospheric pressure and set to pressure of 300 mm Hg.

This technology allows to measure and visualize (through a dedicated software) the distribution of the anal canal pressure at 360° allowing to have a 3D vision of the bowel (Fig. 6.6) [10, 11].

Fig. 6.5 Medtronic single-use sheath with an end tip balloon for 3D catheters

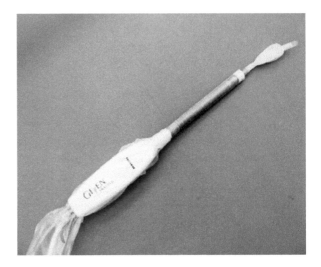

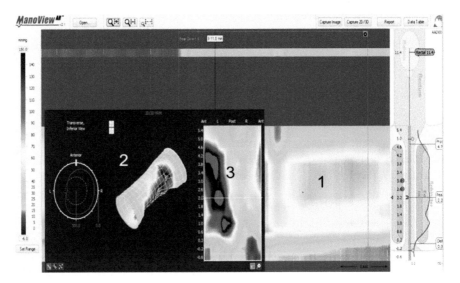

Fig. 6.6 HDMA graphic representation: (1) Classic contour plot visualization where the pressure values shown correspond to the average of the values of each single ring composed of 16 sensors; (2) Display of the pressure values of each of the 256 sensors on the cylinder that represents the catheter. Each rectangle of the grid visible on the cylinder corresponds to a pressure sensor. A more pronounced longitudinal white line on the cylinder indicates the anterior area; (3) Open view on the front of the cylinder: this modality makes clear the mapping and the pressure distribution inside the anal sphincter; it is thus possible to distinguish the four quadrants and also have information on the distance from the distal margin

During the procedure HDAM-3D the probe is kept still and the possible movements of the sphincter during the different phases of the exam can be compensated during the analysis by modifying the position of the markers on the screen. The software is equipped with a tool called eSleeve (electronic sleeve) [10].

In Fig. 6.6, the eSleeve is represented by the two orange dots visible on the right side of the image.

The advantages in the execution of HRAM and HDAM are clearly evident during the preparatory phase of the exam: since no perfusion is necessary, all the time necessary to verify the functioning of all the channels to be perfused is eliminated.

On the other hand, the time taken to sanitize the catheter after each procedure must be considered; indeed, a high-level disinfection of the catheter is required.

Since the sensitivity of solid-state catheters is extraordinarily greater than the corresponding perfused catheters and that the acquisition methodology also changes, standardization protocols of the method and normality values are needed [10–12].

References

1. Jones MP, Post J. High-resolution manometry in the evaluation of anorectal disorders: a simultaneous comparison with water-perfused manometry. Am J Gastroenterol. 2007;102:850–5.
2. Jorge JM, Wexner SD. Anorectal manometry: techniques and clinical applications. South Med J. 1993;86:924–31.
3. Diamant NE, Kamm MA, Wald A, Whitehead WE. AGA technical review on anorectal testing techniques. Gastroenterology. 1999;116:735–60.
4. Carrington EV, Brokjaer A, Craven H, et al. Traditional measures of normal anal sphincter function using high-resolution anorectal manometry (HRAM) in 115 healthy volunteers. Neurogastroenterol Motil. 2014;26:625–35.
5. Jung KW, Joo S, Yang DH, et al. A novel high-resolution anorectal manometry parameter based on a three-dimensional integrated pressurized volume of a spatiotemporal plot, for predicting balloon expulsion in asymptomatic normal individuals. Neurogastroenterol Motil. 2014;26:937–49.
6. Jones MP, Post J, Crowell MD. High-resolution manometry in the evaluation of anorectal disorders: a simultaneous comparison with water-perfused manometry. Am J Gastroenterol. 2007;102:850–5.
7. Lee YY, Erdogan A, Rao SS. High resolution and high definition anorectal manometry and pressure topography: diagnostic advance or a new kid on the block? Curr Gastroenterol Rep. 2013;15:360.
8. Kang HR, Lee JE, Lee JS, et al. Comparison of high-resolution anorectal manometry with water-perfused anorectal manometry. J Neurogastroenterol Motil. 2015;21:126–32.
9. Kang HR, Lee J-E. Comparison of high-resolution anorectal manometry with water-perfused anorectal manometry. J Neurogastroenterol Motil. 2015;21:126–32.
10. Lee TH, Bharucha AE. How to perform and interpret a high-resolution anorectal manometry test. J Neurogastroenterol Motil. 2016;22:46–59.
11. Bredenoord AJ, Hebbard GS. Technical aspects of clinical high-resolution manometry studies. Neurogastroenterol Motil. 2012;24(suppl 1):5–10.
12. Li Y, Yang X. Normal values and pressure morphology for three-dimensional high-resolution anorectal manometry of asymptomatic adults: a study in 110 subjects. Int J Color Dis. 2013;28:1161–8.

Performing, Analyzing, and Interpreting HRAM and HDAM Recordings

7

Edda Battaglia, Lucia D'Alba, Antonella La Brocca, and Francesco Torresan

7.1 Performing HRAM and HDAM

Anorectal manometry is the most widely performed test for the assessment of anal sphincter function and anorectal coordination [1]. Nevertheless, both recording equipment and methodology remain under standardized, which can significantly affect the interpretation of results [2]. The last decade has seen the development of high resolution manometry (HRM) with key improvements being: an increased number of closely spaced micro-transducers greatly enhancing spatial resolution, the ability to measure pressure changes circumferentially, and a software development to allow interpolation between adjacent micro-transducers providing the option of detailed topographical plots of intraluminal pressure events relative to time and location. The preliminary feasibility study evaluating HRM and simultaneously performed conventional water-perfused manometry showed the two methods to be significantly correlated and HRM providing greater resolution of the intraluminal pressure environment of the anorectum [3].

The original version of this chapter was revised. The correction to this chapter can be found at https://doi.org/10.1007/978-3-030-32679-1_11

E. Battaglia (✉)
Physiopatology and Manometry Section, Gastroenterology Unit, Cardinal Massaia Hospital, Asti, Italy

L. D'Alba
Unit of Gastroenterology and Digestive Endoscopy, San Giovanni - Addolorata Hospital, Rome, Italy

A. La Brocca
Department of General and Emergency Surgery, University of Palermo, Palermo, Italy

F. Torresan
Department of Medical and Surgical Sciences, S.Orsola-Malpighi Hospital, University of Bologna, Bologna, Italy

© Springer Nature Switzerland AG 2020
M. Bellini (ed.), *High Resolution and High Definition Anorectal Manometry*,
https://doi.org/10.1007/978-3-030-32419-3_7

The ability to visualize the anorectum as a dynamic structure during test maneuvers should intuitively allow for a better appreciation of normal physiology and hopefully enhance our understanding of the pathophysiology of defecatory dysfunction [4].

HRAM is conducted with water-perfused or solid-state catheters. Water-perfused manometry requires more preparation, technical skills, and training. The dynamic performance of water-perfused systems is several orders of magnitude less than that of solid-state systems, limiting their accuracy when rapidly changing pressures must be measured [5].

One of the principal challenges to adopting HRAM is to establish new normative data sets of an adequate size for recognized measures of anal sphincter function and to promote standardization of the technique, so that results are transferrable between institutions; a problem that has bedeviled traditional practice [2].

The aim of this chapter is making a critical analysis of the fragmented data of the literature and describing the protocol shared by the authors.

7.1.1 Practical Procedure

The procedure with the anorectal high resolution manometry system, described widely in Chap. 6, starts with the clinical evaluation.

A questionnaire assessing study methodology analysis and interpretation of ARM was collected by the International Anorectal Physiology Working Group representing practitioners that perform ARM in Switzerland, UK, and USA. On the basis of various works, it extrapolated that there is marked variation in the methods used to report results of maneuvers, patient preparation, setup, study, and data interpretation [6].

Anorectal manometry is a tertiary test in diagnostic algorithm of fecal incontinence, constipation, and various anorectal diseases. Before manometry, a thorough anamnesis (including chronic diseases, previous surgeries, obstetric traumas, sexual abuses, bowel habit, need for digital disimpaction and/or use of anal dilator, medical systemic and various topical therapy) must be obtained and previous diagnostic tests, eventually performed, must be evaluated (defecography or MR-defecography, transanal, and transrectal ultrasound, etc.).

Ongoing procedure should be explained in every detail in order to render the patient conscious and more collaborative; this makes it possible to perform a more reliable exam.

Most centers execute manometry studies without a written consent form because the procedure poses a minimal risk to patients. However, theoretically the graded balloon distension during the test, although gently carried out, can cause a rectal injury, especially in patients who have previously undergone rectal surgery [7]. Moreover vagal crisis could be elicited. For these reasons the authors usually require informed consent to the procedure.

The exact manometry protocols will vary by center, but generally, the procedure must include an assessment of rectoanal pressure and anal canal length at rest, rectoanal pressures during squeeze, simulated evacuation, and coughing, and rectal sensation. A rectal balloon expulsion test, which is an effective screening test to identify defecatory disorders, should be performed at the same visit as the anorectal manometry [8] (Table 7.1).

Table 7.1 Patient's preparation

1. Continue medications
2. Fasting is not necessary
3. Cleaning enema at least 30 min before the test

7.1.2 Patient Preparation

Patients may continue with their routine medications but the medications should be documented to facilitate interpretation of the data. Topical therapy (nifedipine, lidocaine, etc.) must be stopped 1 day before exam, in order not to influence the anal pressure.

Some authors recommended to avoid food since the night before the exam while others allow patients consuming normal meals [9].

Bowel preparation is optional. Many authors do not require it, but the patients are only asked to empty their bowel before the test. If the digital rectal examination, performed immediately before the manometry, reveals that the rectum is loaded with stool, then a 250–500-mL tap water enema is suggested. In this case, at least 30 min should elapse between evacuation of stool and probe placement [10].

Since the presence of feces in rectal ampoule could modify the results, in order to achieve a better standardization of the test, we suggest all patients performing a cleaning enema in the morning of the HRAM/HDAM at least 30 min before the exam.

7.1.3 Patient Position

The test should be conducted in a quiet room in the presence of strictly necessary personnel, in order to create a relaxed and confident relationship with the patient. It is recommended that the patient is placed in the left lateral position with knees and hips bent to 90° angle (Sims position), to guarantee privacy and discretion to the patient [2].

7.1.4 Digital Examination

As reported above, prior to the catheter insertion, a digital rectal examination should be performed using a lubricated gloved finger (any lubricant to aid probe placement should be non-anesthetizing). The presence of tenderness, stool, or blood on the finger glove should be noted [2]. The digital rectal examination is important to teach the patient the maneuvers to be performed during the exam and to test the ability of the subject to understand the commands "squeeze" and "push" [11]. The authors strongly believe that performing a carefully digital rectal examination before anorectal manometry is necessary and positively influence the outcome of the test.

7.1.5 Probe Placement

The probe is calibrated immediately before the procedure by placing it in a calibration chamber, where it is zeroed to atmospheric pressure and set to a range of pressure up to 300 mmHg. All systems require thermal compensation to correct for the pressure drift with time [10]. After calibrating the instrument, the lubricated probe is gently inserted into the rectum with its dorsal side orientated such that the most distal sensor (1 cm level) is located posteriorly at 1 cm from the anal verge. Once positioned, the probe has to be maintained in the same position for the duration of the test. However it is important to continuously monitor it and the operator has to be aware of possible probe movements, especially after the patient performs maneuvers such as squeeze, cough, or bearing down, and eventually to adjust the position of the probe when necessary.

7.1.6 Test Procedure

The exact manometry protocols vary by center. The procedure must include an assessment of rectoanal pressure and anal canal length at rest, the presence of the cough reflex test, the recording of rectoanal pressures during squeeze, simulated evacuation, coughing, and the evaluation of the rectal sensations. A rectal balloon expulsion test, which is an effective screening test to identify defecatory disorders, should be performed at the end of the anorectal manometry [10] (Table 7.2).

7.1.6.1 Rest
Resting anal pressures must be measured with the subject relaxed, lying still and not speaking during the examination. There is no agreement how long to wait after inserting the probe before beginning the examination. Several laboratory manuals and guidelines recommend waiting for 5 minutes after inserting the probe before taking. One justification for this is the presence of ultraslow wave activity, which might interfere with the interpretation of the resting pressure [2] (Fig. 7.1).

However, there is no scientific basis for the duration of the rest period. A prolonged procedure causes discomfort and reduces the patient compliance. In some patients, anorectal manometry can cause pain and discomfort [12]. Dakshitha Praneeth Wickramasinghe et al. analyzing data from 100 consecutive patients who

Table 7.2 Test procedure

Resting anal pressure: sphincteric length, resting pressure
Cough reflex test
Squeeze pressure and squeeze duration
Push
RAIR rectoanal inhibitory reflex
Rectal compliance
Rectal volume tolerability (first sensation, urge to defecate and discomfort volume)

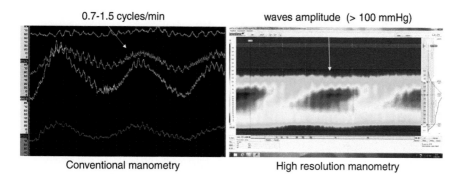

Fig. 7.1 Ultraslow waves

underwent HDAM found that 99% of the patients had their anal canal resting pressure stabilize in <150 s. Therefore a standard ARM assessment can be completed in several minutes. Since there were no significant associations between sex or the age and the time taken for the pressure to stabilize, the waiting time can be recommended for all adult patients, irrespective of their age or sex.

We think that a 1 min wait before starting the recording is sufficient to allow the anal resting pressure to stabilize in the most patients, waiting more time (3 min) only in the presence of ultraslow wave activity. The resting pressure must be recorded at least three times for 1 min, in order to allow a statistically significant average to be carried out.

7.1.6.2 Cough Reflex Test
This maneuver is indicated to assess the integrity of spinal reflex pathways between the rectum and anal canal in patients with incontinence. The patient is asked to cough. Normally, the increased abdominal pressure triggers external sphincter contraction. The maneuver is repeated once more after 10 s [2].

7.1.7 Squeeze

Squeeze pressure is the difference between the maximum voluntary pressure during squeeze contraction and the resting pressure at the same level of the anal canal. The patient is asked to squeeze the anus as long as possible, for a maximum of 30 s, followed by a 30 s rest. *Sphincter endurance* is the length of time that the patient can maintain a squeeze pressure above the resting pressure.

By convention, this maneuver is performed three times. In the unusual event of poor participant compliance a further attempt is allowed at the practitioner's discretion.

Ideally rectal pressure should not increase because that would imply that the patient has contracted the abdominal wall [10] (Fig. 7.2).

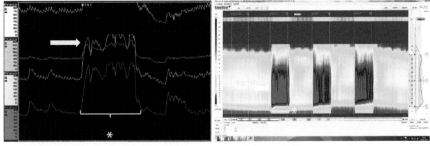

Conventional anorectal manometry   High resolution anorectal manometry

Fig. 7.2 Squeeze pressure. Squeeze pressure: the highest pressure during maximal contraction of anal sphincter (white arrow). Squeeze duration: the longest interval, in seconds, between the onset of increase in anal sphincter pressure and when this pressure returned to baseline value (*)

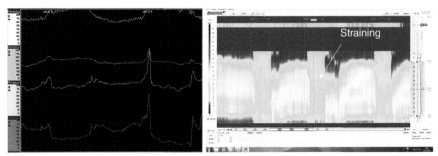

Conventional anorectal manometry   High resolution anorectal manometry

Fig. 7.3 Straining maneuver. Assessment of pressure changes during simulated evacuation. Discoordination of abdominal, rectoanal, and pelvic floor muscles

7.1.8   Simulated Defecation

The patient is asked to bear down as if to defecate. This test is conducted inflating 5 mL of air in the rectal balloon, and pushes down for 30 s and is repeated for three times separated by a 30 s interval. It is essential to instruct patients to not withhold the probe. Indeed, coaching patients while they perform maneuvers might enhance the accuracy of the test. In one study, coaching changed the diagnosis based on manometry from "pathologic" to "normal" values in 14 of 31 patients with incontinence and in 12 of 39 patients with dyssynergic defecation [13] (Fig. 7.3).

7.1.9   RAIR (Rectoanal Inhibitory Reflex)

This maneuver examines the integrity of the myenteric plexus between rectum and anal canal. This maneuver consists of intermittent balloon distension in the rectum to assess the relaxation of the internal anal sphincter, while the RAIR can generally

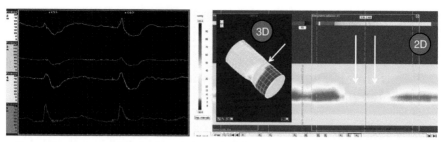

Conventional anorectal manometry

High Definition anorectal manometry: white arrows shows the decrease of pressure after inflating the rectal balloon, both in 2D and 3D.

Fig. 7.4 RAIR Rectoanal inhibitory reflex. This maneuver examines the integrity of the myenteric plexus between the rectum and anal canal

be elicited just by a volume of 20 mL of air. Repeating the maneuver for three times, using increasing volumes up to 60–80 mL, it is sufficient to properly assess the presence and the quality of the reflex. If no RAIR is recorded, the following measures may solve the problem: (1) ask the patient not to contract the external anal sphincter during rectal distension, (2) make sure there is no fecal impaction, and (3) increase the rectal distension up to a maximum volume of 250 mL to exclude acquired megarectum [10] (Fig. 7.4).

7.1.10 Rectal Sensation, Graded Balloon Distension

Evaluation of rectal sensation is performed by inflating the balloon placed at the tip of catheter in the rectum. The increasing distension allows to assess the rectal sensation which can be classified as follows:

– *Sensory threshold*: is the minimum rectal volume perceived by the patient.
– *Urge sensation*: is the volume associated with the initial urge to defecate.
– *Maximum tolerated volume*: is the volume at which the patient experiences discomfort and an uncontrollable desire to defecate.

To assess rectal sensation, the rectal balloon is initially distended with air with increments of 10 mL, until the patient reports a first sensation. Thereafter, the balloon is increased in 20 mL steps to a maximum volume of 400 mL. The distension should be ended earlier if the maximum tolerable volume is reached. Each distension is maintained for at least 30 s. *Rectal compliance* (i.e., pressure-volume relationships) can also be measured during balloon distension but the rectal balloon used for HRAM and HDAM is relatively stiff. For example, when the given HRM catheter balloon is inflated by 50 mL in atmosphere, it has a pressure of 137 mmHg. In theory, rectal compliance can be estimated by subtracting this pressure from the measured balloon pressure during rectal distention. However, in general, rectal compliance measured with an anorectal manometry is not as accurate as measurements obtained with a barostat [10].

7.2 Normal Values for High Resolution Anorectal Manometry

Prior to the introduction of HRM catheters in 2007, anorectal manometry was performed with non-high resolution, water-perfused, or solid-state catheters. Since then HRAM and HDAM catheters are increasingly used in clinical practice, but the long-standing problem of the normality values of traditional ARM is still the biggest problem for a widespread clinical application of this new technique, at least for its use in the study of anorectal pathophysiology.

In addition, anal sphincter pressures at rest and during anal contraction (i.e., squeeze maneuver) recorded with HRAM and conventional ARM are significantly correlated but they tend to be higher when measured with HRAM [14–16]. The rectoanal pressure gradient measured with both techniques was also strongly correlated but the gradient was more negative when evaluated with conventional ARM (−66 mmHg) than with HRAM [16].

Several small studies have evaluated the normal values of HRAM and HDAM [10]. Carrington et al. [11] assess diagnostic accuracy of HRAM in comparison with conventional ARM in terms of discriminating patients with fecal incontinence (FI) vs healthy volunteers (HV). Asymptomatic female volunteers were selected without constipation (Cleveland Clinic Constipation Score, CCCS < 9 [17]) or incontinence (St Marks Incontinence Score, SMIS < 6 [18]), current or previous significant gastrointestinal disease [19], functional gastrointestinal symptoms, previous anal or pelvic surgery, pregnancy or lactation [20], without history of diabetes, cardiovascular, renal, or hepatic disease. In the standard method using (UniTip; UniSensor AG, Attikon, Switzerland) of 12 F external diameter incorporating 12 micro-transducers and using commercially available manometric system (Solar GI HRM v9.1; MMS/Laborie, Enschede, Netherlands) (Table 7.3).

The authors acknowledge a number of limitations of this study: the first one is that it included only female participants and this, naturally, limits the application of assumptions to men. Although it was assumed that all healthy participants had normal anal sphincter function, even if 49/85 HVs were parous, the effect of vaginal delivery on sphincter function is well-documented. No assessment of sphincter anatomy was performed, and if extrapolated from previous studies, between 11% and 27% [21] of parous volunteers would be anticipated to have a degree of external sphincter damage. Matching of HV and FI groups for age and parity was suboptimal; however, data for the effect of age and parity on sphincter function in health are conflicting [11].

The data are certainly not convincing and conclusive. For example, it should be noted that the normal range of anal pressures is relatively wide: from 33 to 91 mmHg among women aged >50 years in one study with HRAM [21].

Table 7.3 HR-manometry and 3D-high resolution manometry measures in healthy women and men (from Lee et al. [10], Cross-Adame et al. [9], Carrington et al. [11])

	Healthy Women						Healthy Men	
	Rest		Squeeze					Rest
	HR-ARM-RP mmHgcm30 s	3DHRAM	HR-ARM-SI mmHg	HR-ARM-SP mmHgcm5 s	3DHRAM			HR-ARM-RP mmHgcm30
Mean	163	76.6	122	368	148		Mean	73
							95%CI	56.5–65.5
Median	151	95.6	112	342	180		Median	46
SD	71	30.3	64	194	72		SD	23
Minimum	67	43	20	45	171		Minimum	94
Maximum	408	86	291	868	190		Maximum	732

HR-ARM-RP high resolution manometry resting pressure, *3DHRAM* three dimensional high resolution manometry, *HR-ARM-SI* high resolution anorectal manometry squeeze increment, *HR-ARM-SP* high resolution anorectal manometry squeeze pressure

In asymptomatic women, the HPZ is, on average, 3.5 cm long, and not correlated with age [22]. In one study, a longer HPZ was associated with a specific phenotype among patients with defecatory disorders [22]. Intuitively, a longer HPZ probably reflects a more effective continence mechanism. However, further studies are required to assess the utility of measuring the dimensions of the HPZ for discriminating between healthy people and patients with fecal incontinence.

However, because the sample size in these studies was relatively small, additional studies are necessary to define more precisely the normal range for HRAM and HDAM.

Squeeze pressures are lower in women than men and in older than younger people [11, 21–23]. Hence, normal values are stratified by age and sex. The absolute squeeze pressure and the change from the resting pressure should be considered when interpreting the test.

In a large cohort of patients with functional anorectal disorders the results of 3D high resolution anorectal manometry (3DHRAM) provide reference values for 3DHRAM in patients with functional anorectal disorders [24].

At the current state of the art, it is really difficult to provide data of shared normality between different centers performing HRAM/HDAM and the data provided in the various studies can only represent a generic guide to the various operators. To have validated data it will be necessary to wait for an international consensus based on large multicenter studies. Therefore, at present it is suggested that each motility center creates its own set of normality.

7.3 Which Diagnosis?

HRAM and HDAM are functional exams that can help the clinicians to reach the right diagnosis on different anorectal disorders, functional and anatomic, and to tailor the treatment on the patient.

The functional anorectal disorders can be divided, according to Roma IV criteria, into three categories: (1) fecal incontinence, (2) functional anorectal pain ((a) levator ani syndrome, (b) unspecified functional anorectal pain, (c) proctalgia fugax), (3) functional defecation disorders ((a) inadequate defecatory propulsion, (b) dyssynergic defecation) [1].

The groups that can benefit from the use of HRAM and HDAM in the diagnostic process are the first one and the third one.

7.4 Fecal Incontinence

According to the Roma IV criteria, fecal incontinence (FI) is the uncontrolled passage of solid or liquid stool that occurs at least two times in a 4-week period with no distinction made on the basis of presumed etiology (functional, structural, or neurological) [2]. Endoanal ultrasound (EAUS) is the gold standard for detecting anal sphincter defects in patients with (FI), while anorectal manometry evaluates sphincter function [25]. A recent study cohort that included 39 patients with FI shows that 21 patients had an anal sphincter defect on EAUS with a median size of 93° (range 40–136°). Fourteen (36%) had a defect shown by HDAM. The sensitivity, specificity, and positive and negative predictive values of HDAM in detecting a sphincter defect were 75%, 74%, 43%, and 92%, respectively. Then, with a negative predictive value of 92%, HDAM could be a useful screening method for ruling out a sphincter defect in patients with FI, thereby avoiding both EAUS and manometry in selected patients [26]. HRAM or HDAM is then not necessary for the diagnosis but they are useful for a more precise evaluation of FI. Identifying a weakness of the internal anal sphincter (with an anal resting pressure below the normal level, common in the passive FI) or/and of the external anal sphincter (with a pressure during voluntary squeeze effort below the normal level, common in the FI with urgency) allows clinicians to address the patients toward the most suitable treatment and to a quantitative evaluation of the effects of their treatments (Fig. 7.5).

HDAM is also useful in the diagnostic process of iatrogenic FI due to previous surgery. The HDAM is more recommended than HRAM in these cases, because only HDAM is able to identify the exact localization of the damage (anterior, posterior, left or right side of the anal canal). An endoanal ultrasound is obviously mandatory to confirm the diagnosis.

A typical example is FI after the left lateral internal sphincterotomy for the treatment of a chronic anal fissure. If the internal anal sphincter has been damaged, while recording the resting pressure, it is easy to see a reduced resting tone of the left side of the anal canal, where the sphincterotomy has been performed. If the external anal sphincter has also been damaged during the same procedure a reduced tone of the left side of the anal canal is detectable during the squeezing.

Also patients that undergo low anterior resection for treating a rectal cancer can develop incontinence. In this case the incontinence is due to a nervous damage of the sacral plexus, rather than a direct damage on the sphincters and therefore HDAM could be less specific and useful [5].

HDAM plays also an important role in postpartum (after vaginal delivery) FI which could be due to third-degree anal sphincter tear [6], or to obstetric injury to the pudendal nerve [7]. The right diagnosis can help in choosing the treatment. HDAM, instead of HRAM, is recommended also in these cases, to differentiate an anal sphincter tear, that is characterized by a generalized weakness of all the sphincter apparatus.

7.5 Functional Defecation Disorders

Inadequate defecatory propulsion and dyssynergic defecation can be well identified by both HRAM and HDAM.

(a) The *inadequate defecatory propulsion* is the impaired rectal force during simulated defecation. If the patient is affected by inadequate defecatory propulsion, the normal increment of pressure (at least 40–45 mmHg more than the resting pres-

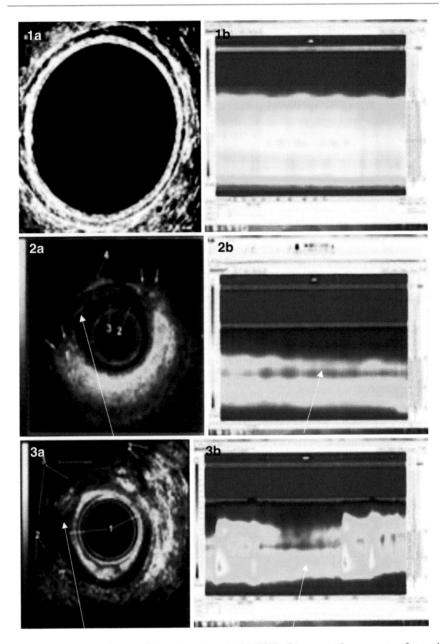

Fig. 7.5 Fecal incontinence. Normal canal anal: (**a**) EUS, (**b**) anorectal manometry. Internal sphincter lesion: (**c**) EUS, (**d**) anorectal manometry. External sphincter lesion: (**e**) EUS, (**f**) anorectal manometry

sure) recorded by the sensor located in the rectal ampulla is not visualized during the phase of ~~squeezing~~ push straining. In this condition, the relaxation of the sphincter is normal during the simulated defecation. The inadequate defecatory propulsion is common in old patients, because the weakness of the abdominal wall cannot produce the force necessary for the act of defecation, so even if the sphincters are relaxed, there is no propulsive force for pushing out the stools [1].

(b) *Dyssynergic defecation* is characterized by a paradoxical contraction or an inability to relax the anal sphincter and/or puborectalis muscle; or impaired abdominal and rectal pushing forces. It has been classified by Rao et al. into four types, in relationship to the pressure developed by the abdominal wall and the sphincter tone. In the first type the abdominal pressure is present, but the sphincter is not able to relax [1]; in the second type, the sphincter contracts itself instead of relax, with a paradoxical contraction; in the third type, the manometric pattern shows a weak or absent abdominal pressure; in the fourth type, there is also an unrelaxed or contracted sphincter [8] (Fig. 7.6).

The presence of a *paradoxical contraction* is defined as an increase in sphincter pressure >40 mmHg, confirmed by a negative percentage of anal relaxation and a negative *defecation index (or rectoanal pressure gradient)* defined as a ratio of intrarectal pressure/anal residual pressure.

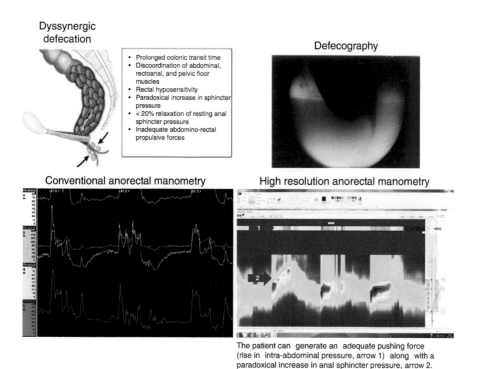

The patient can generate an adequate pushing force (rise in intra-abdominal pressure, arrow 1) along with a paradoxical increase in anal sphincter pressure, arrow 2.

Fig. 7.6 Dyssynergic defecation

Impaired anal sphincter relaxation is defined as absent decrease or a decrease <20% in anal sphincter pressure [9].

HRAM and HDAM can better detect than conventional ARM the presence of dyssynergia because the probe contemporarily records the pressures into the rectal ampulla and into the anal canal. The other exam providing the same *contemporary* assessment of the defecation is defecography (MRI/RX), but the evaluated parameters are different, so they can be considered complementary exams.

7.6 Anatomical Abnormalities

Anorectal abnormalities such as rectal intussusception and rectal prolapse, rectocele, descending perineum syndrome can be detected with HRAM and HDAM, even if the radiological imaging remains the "gold standard."

Rectal prolapse by HRAM can be hypothesized by an increase in the pressure above the high pressure zone (corresponding to the anal canal) evident during the first straining to evacuate, more clear at the second attempt, and glaring to the eye's investigator at the third (Fig. 7.7).

In the HDAM the presence of a rectal prolapse is hypothesized by the presence of an increase in pressure around the probe with straining to evacuate, exactly such as something is rolling on the probe. The pressure pattern findings are a decreased resting tone as well as decreased squeeze pressures, with 40% of patients with rectal prolapse demonstrating incompetent sphincters [23].

The *rectocele with anal intussusception* can be detected by an increased rectal pressure with a narrow band of high pressure within the anal canal during simulated defecation [27]. The *descending perineum syndrome* is characterized

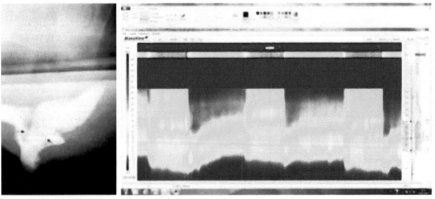

Defecography   High resolution anorectal manometry

Fig. 7.7 Rectal prolapse. Defecography, which is performed in a sitting position usually aids diagnosis in patients who report prolapse. Anorectal manometry may reveal low resting sphincter pressure especially in patients with complete rectal prolapse, rectal sensation and compliance may be impaired. Pre-existing dyssynergic defecation that causes chronic excessive straining may coexist

by the perineal descent on the manometric probe during the attempted defecation, with the regaining by the perineum of the initial position at the end of the bear down [28].

Even if the diagnosis of these anatomical changes remains radiological, however it is really important to add a functional exam like HRAM/HDAM, where available, since the acquisition of the morphological elements associated with the functional ones is the most complete way to evaluate the alteration of the defecatory function.

It is already known that anatomical abnormalities, such as a rectal prolapse, may be the result of a hidden dyssynergic defecation. The excessive straining that characterizes the dyssynergic defecation generally leads to a laxity of the connective tissue and to a nervous damage, ending into the opposite problem which is FI [29]. We strongly suggest to perform a HRAM/HDAM in a patient with rectal prolapse as well as rectocele, solitary rectal ulcer syndrome, and descending perineum syndrome, because the chronic excessive straining due to a pre-existing dyssynergic defecation may be the reason why the patient has developed an anatomical defect, so the surgical correction of the defect will be incomplete or ineffective if the underlying cause persists. It is worth emphasizing that in the rectal prolapse it is advisable to carry out the manual reduction of the prolapse itself before performing the test.

The importance of discovering functional abnormalities in these patients is very clear looking at a surgical setting. For example, if the patient with rectal prolapse is a candidate for surgery, the laxity of pelvic floor and of the connective tissue relates to the continuous straining consequent to the obstructed defecation might lead to a subsequent FI.

Sometimes the evidence of an underlying dyssynergic defecation, or the evidence of a pre-existing reduced sphincter tone, cannot modify the surgical planning, but it has a prognostic value; and the patient could perform a preoperative biofeedback to improve the performance of the pelvic floor and to ensure a better quality of postsurgical continence.

7.7 Hirschsprung's Disease

Hirschsprung's disease is a genetic disease due to the congenital absence of ganglion cells in the distal bowel, with the most prominent symptom of constipation. The suspect is clinical, shortly after birth, because of the presence of megacolon, or because the baby fails to pass the meconium in 48 h of delivery [30].

The diagnostic route of Hirschsprung includes HRAM and rectal suction biopsy. HDAM is not used in children, because of the diameter of the probe.

This disease is characterized by the lack of the rectoanal inhibitory reflex (RAIR), and this can be detected by the HRAM, because, since the distal colon is dilated, the reflex cannot be elicited by the rectal balloon (Fig. 7.8).

The lack of the RAIR is not always so obvious, this is why has been identified a new parameter to assist the diagnosis of Hirschsprung's disease: The ASRI10, i.e., "anal sphincter relaxation integral" at pressure cutoff <10 mmHg. It is

Rectal biopsy: absence   3D-HR Manometry: absence of RAIR
of ganglion cells

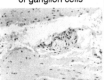

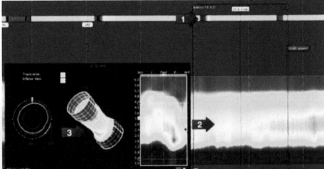

Abdominal radiograph:
megacolon

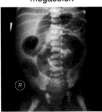

Even after ten balloon filling maneuvers (maximum air insufflations 240cc)
(arrow 1), no rectal-anal inhibitory reflex is appreciated on the sphincterial
sensors, with permanence of the HPZ on the 2D colour-contour plot
(arrow 2) and reduced caliber on the 3D reconstruction (arrow 3).

Radiograph after water
soluble contrast enema:
megarectum

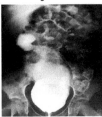

Fig. 7.8 Hirschsprung's disease

present in the automatic HRAM analysis system, and can quantify the *RAIR adequacy*. A complete discussion about ASRI10 is beyond the aim of this chapter [31].

In conclusion, if the RAIR is present, Hirschsprung's disease can be ruled out. On the other hand, if the RAIR is absent, rectal suction biopsy is mandatory. This is the reason because some clinicians prefer to use only the rectal suction biopsy, but, using HRAM as first choice diagnostic test can reduce the number of patients undergoing an invasive procedure like rectal biopsy [32].

References

1. Cott SM, Gladman MA. Manometric, sensorimotor, and europhysiologic evaluation of anorectal function. Gastroenterol Clin N Am. 2008;37:511–38.
2. Rao SS, Azpiroz F, Diamant N, Enck P, Tougas G, Wald A. Minimum standards of anorectal manometry. Neurogastroenterol Motil. 2002;14:553–9.
3. Jones MP, Post J, Crowell MD. High-resolution manometry in the evaluation of anorectal disorders: simultaneous comparison with water-perfused manometry. Am J Gastroenterol. 2007;102:850–5.

4. Ratuapli SK, Bharucha AE, Noelting J, Harvey DM, Zinsmeister AR. Pheno-typic identification and classification of functional defecatory disorders using high-resolution anorectal manometry. Gastroenterology. 2012;144:314–22.
5. Bredenoord AJ, Hebbard GS. Technical aspects of clinical high-resolution manometry studies. Neurogastroenterol Motil. 2012;24(suppl 1):5–10.
6. Carrington EV, Heinrich H, Knowles CH, Rao SS, Fox M, Scott SM. International anorectal physiology working party group (IAPWG). Methods of anorectal manometry vary widely in clinical practice: results from an international survey. Neurogastroenterol Motil. 2017;29(8):e13016.
7. Azpiroz F, Enck P, Whitehead WE. Anorectal functional testing: review of collective experience. Am J Gastroenterol. 2002;97:232–40.
8. Wald A, Bharucha AE, Cosman BC, Whitehead WE. ACG clinical guideline: management of benign anorectal disorders. Am J Gastroenterol. 2014;109:1141–57.
9. Cross-Adame E, Rao SS, Valestin J, Ali-Azamar A, Remes-Troche JM. Accuracy and reproducibility of high-definition anorectal manometry and pressure topography analyses in healthy subjects. Clin Gastroenterol Hepatol. 2015;13(6):1143–50.
10. Lee TH, Barucha A. How to perform and interpret a high-resolution anorectal manometry test. J Neurogastreoenterol Motil. 2016;22:46–59.
11. Carrington EV, Brokjaer A, Craven H, et al. Traditional measures of normal anal sphincter function using high-resolution anorectal manometry (HRAM) in 115 healthy volunteers. Neurogastroenterol Motil. 2014;26:625–35.
12. Szojda MM, et al. Referral for anorectal function evaluation is indicated in 65% and beneficial in 92% of patients. World J Gastroenterol. 2008;14(2):272–7.
13. Heinrich H, Fruehauf H, Sauter M, et al. The effect of standard compared to enhanced instruction and verbal feedback on anorectal manometry measurements. Neurogastroenterol Motil. 2013;25:230–7, e163.
14. Jones MP, Post J, Crowell MD. High-resolution manometry in the evaluation of anorectal disorders: a simultaneous comparison with waterperfused manometry. Am J Gastroenterol. 2007;102:850–5.
15. Sauter M, Heinrich H, Fox M, et al. Toward more accurate measurements of anorectal motor and sensory function in routine clinical practice: validation of high-resolution anorectal manometry and Rapid Barostat Bag measurements of rectal function. Neurogastroenterol Motil. 2014;26:685–95.
16. Lee YY, Erdogan A, Rao SS. High resolution and high definition anorectal manometry and pressure topography: diagnostic advance or a new kid on the block? Curr Gastroenterol Rep. 2013;15:360.
17. Agachan F, Chen T, Pfeifer J, et al. A constipation scoring system to simplify evaluation and management of constipated patients. Dis Colon Rectum. 1996;39:681–5.
18. Vaizey CJ, Carapeti E, Cahill JA, et al. Prospective comparison of faecal incontinence grading systems. Gut. 1999;44:77–80.
19. Longstreth GF, Thompson WG, Chey WD, et al. Functional bowel disorders. Gastroenterology. 2006;130:1480–91.
20. Dudding TC, Vaizey CJ, Kamm MA. Obstetric anal sphincter injury: incidence, risk factors, and management. Ann Surg. 2008;247:224–37.
21. Noelting J, Ratuapli SK, Bharucha AE, Harvey DM, Ravi K, Zinsmeister AR. Normal values for high-resolution anorectal manometry in healthy women: effects of age and significance of rectoanal gradient. Am J Gastroenterol. 2012;107:1530–6.
22. Ratuapli SK, Bharucha AE, Noelting J, Harvey DM, Zinsmeister AR. Phenotypic identification and classification of functional defecatory disorders using high-resolution anorectal manometry. Gastroenterology. 2013;144:314–22.
23. Hotouras A, Murphy J, Boyle DJ, Allison M, Williams NS, Chan CL. Assessment of female patients with rectal intussusception and prolapse: is this a progressive spectrum of disease? Dis Colon Rectum. 2013;56(6):780–5.

24. Andrianjafy C, Luciano L, Bazin C, Baumstarck K, Bouvier M, Vitton V. Three-dimensional high-resolution anorectal manometry in functional anorectal disorders: results from a large observational cohort study. Int J Color Dis. 2019;34:719–29.
25. Dakshitha PW, Umesh J, Dharmabandhu NS. Duration taken for the anal sphincter pressures to stabilize prior to anorectal manometry. BMC Research Notes. 2018;11(354).
26. Rezaie A, Iriana S, Pimentel M, Murrell Z, Fleshner P, Zaghiyan K. Can three-dimensional high-resolution anorectal manometry detect anal sphincter defects in patients with faecal incontinence? Color Dis. 2017;19(5):468–75.
27. Heinrich H, Sauter M, Fox M, Weishaupt D, Halama M, Misselwitz B, Buetikofer S, Reiner C, Fried M, Schwizer W, Fruehauf H. Assessment of obstructive defecation by high-resolution anorectal manometry compared with magnetic resonance defecography. Clin Gastroenterol Hepatol. 2015;13:1310–7.
28. Vitton V, Grimaud JC, Bouvier M. Three-dimension high-resolution anorectal manometry can precisely measure perineal descent. J Neurogastroenterol Motil. 2013;19(2):257–8.
29. Patcharatrakul T, Rao SSC. Update on the pathophysiology and management of anorectal disorders. Gut Liver. 2018;12(4):375–84.
30. Moore SW. Advances in understanding functional variations in the Hirschsprung disease spectrum (variant Hirschsprung disease). Pediatr Surg Int. 2017;33(3):285–98.
31. Wu JF, Lu CH, Yang CH, Tsai IJ. Diagnostic role of anal sphincter relaxation integral in high-resolution anorectal manometry for Hirschsprung disease in infants. J Pediatr. 2018;194:136–41.
32. Meinds RJ, Trzpis M, Broen PMA. Anorectal manometry may reduce the number of rectal suction biopsy procedures needed to diagnose Hirschsprung disease. J Pediatr Gastroenterol Nutr. 2018;67(3):322–7.

High-Resolution Anorectal Manometry and 3D High-Definition Anorectal Manometry in Pediatric Settings

8

Teresa Di Chio, Marcella Pesce, Diego Peroni, and Osvaldo Borrelli

8.1 Anorectal Physiology

Fecal continence and defecation are highly regulated processes ensured by the synergic and coordinated function of the rectum, pelvic floor muscles, and anal canal. The rectum functions as a reservoir for fecal material and its stretch-sensitive fibers, activated by the intraluminal distension, are essential in signaling the awareness of defecation to the central nervous system and activating spinal reflexes. The anal canal consists of the internal (IAS) and external (EAS) anal sphincters. The former, which is composed of smooth muscle cells, is innervated by the enteric nervous system and therefore not under voluntary control. It is primarily responsible for anal continence as it generates approximately 70–85% of the anal canal pressure. Conversely, the EAS, composed by skeletal muscle cells, is under the voluntary control of the sacral nerves. The two sphincters are closely adjoined and, in young children, a clear physical separation between is difficult to detect [1, 2].

The anal sphincters, the pelvic floor muscles, and the levator ani complex, which includes the puborectalis muscle, are responsible for ensuring the fecal continence at rest. Synergistically, through tonic contractions, the aforementioned structures maintain the anorectum angulated between 85° and 105° [3] and generate a pressure at the level of anal canal that exceeds the rectal pressure, hence preventing the involuntary loss of fecal material [3, 4].

T. Di Chio · D. Peroni
Department of Clinical and Experimental Medicine, Section of Pediatric, University of Pisa, Pisa, Italy

M. Pesce
Department of Gastroenterology, GI Physiology Unit, University College London Hospitals, London, UK

O. Borrelli (✉)
Department of Gastroenterology, Division of Neurogastroenterology and Motility, Great Ormond Street Hospital, London, UK
e-mail: osvaldo.borrelli@gosh.nhs.uk.

© Springer Nature Switzerland AG 2020
M. Bellini (ed.), *High Resolution and High Definition Anorectal Manometry*,
https://doi.org/10.1007/978-3-030-32419-3_8

97

The evacuatory process is a highly regulated and voluntary function. The distension of the rectal wall above an appropriate sensory threshold provokes a temporary reflex relaxation of the IAS, named recto-anal inhibitory reflex (RAIR), which enables the luminal contents to enter the anal canal. The expulsive step, under voluntary control, is characterized by the coordinated relaxation of the EAS and pelvic floor muscles alongside with the abdominal wall contraction, which ultimately enables the passage of the stools through the anal canal [4]. If the subject is not in a socially appropriate setting to defecate, the voluntary contraction of the EAS and the puborectalis muscle prevent the defecation and the stools are returned to the colon by reverse peristalsis.

8.2 Equipment

ARM is by nature a highly technical evaluation and when knowledgeably used, provides an accurate description of anorectal neuromuscular function. However, the manometric data are reliable only if the methodology used to acquire them is accurate.

A manometric apparatus setup consists of a pressure sensor/transducer combination, which detects the pressures in the anal canal and rectum and transduces them into an electrical signal, and a recording device, which amplifies, records, and stores that electrical signal. The pressure sensor/transducer components of the manometric assembly function as a matched pair and are available in two general designs: either water-perfused catheters, connected to a pneumohydraulic perfusion pump and to volume displacement transducers, or strain gauge transducers with solid state circuitry [5].

In the last decade considerable advancements in ARM technology have been witnessed and conventional low-resolution systems have gradually been replaced by high-resolution (HRARM) and 3D high-definition manometry (HDARM). This has been achieved by a combination of new manometric assemblies allowing intraluminal pressure to be recorded from up to 256 pressure sensors spaced <0.3 mm. At the same time, advances in computer processing allow pressure data to be presented in real-time as a compact, either as two-dimensional visually intuitive "spatiotemporal plot" or more sophisticated 3D. In adults, by correlating with anatomic structures defined by MRI or 3D ultrasound, HDARM measurements allow a better definition of the contribution of different components of the anal canal and a better description of the anal canal radial asymmetry [6]. However, the role of our enhanced knowledge of the pathophysiological mechanisms of the different defecation disorders in children is still unclear.

Currently, the catheter used for 3DHRAM has an outer diameter of almost 11 mm [7]. Although the test could in theory be performed at any age, in infants the anal resting pressure could be overestimated and anal canal dynamics upon balloon distension could be misinterpreted [8]. To date, 3DHRAM has been used in children aged above 2 years.

8.3   Methodological Aspects

8.3.1   Preparation of Pediatric Patients and Caregivers

In preparation for the procedure, in children above the age of 1 year, an enema is recommended on the day or the evening prior to the day of tests. Alternatively, in those with significant fecal loading a degree of bowel preparation could be required prior to the procedure. In infants, no bowel preparation is required as they generally have soft stools [9]. Medications that can interfere with the anorectal function should be stopped before the procedure.

Older children are instructed to defecate if required before the test. The child should be placed in the lateral decubitus position, with knees drawn up to the chest, maintaining the hips and knees flexed at 90°. Before the probe insertion, the perianal area should be inspected and a digital rectal examination should be carried out, in order to evaluate the general anatomy, the perianal sensation, skin excoriation, and the presence of rectal impaction. Then, the lubricated manometry probe can be gently inserted into the rectum. Before starting the recording, the operator should wait for few minutes in order to allow the acclimation of anorectal area.

Pediatric gastroenterologists have often to face non-cooperative children and, especially in children under the age of 5, a study under anesthesia may be required. When that happens, only the analysis of anal sphincter resting pressures and RAIR can be performed. Moreover, the results need to be carefully evaluated as different anesthetic agents may interfere with the physiological outcomes [10–13].

Nevertheless, in some circumstances and indications undoubtedly requiring patients' cooperation a proper psychological preparation for both children and parents is certainly required. Anorectal manometry has been shown to induce significant preprocedural distress in children and adequate psychological preparation intervention has been shown to reduce anticipatory distress, to improve measurements reliability, and ultimately to better pave future treatments based on the manometric patterns [12, 14–17].

8.3.2   Study Protocol, Analysis, and Interpretation

Ideally, the full manometric protocol should aim at assessing sphincter pressures at rest and during voluntary contractions, bear-down maneuvers, rectal sensation, and reflexes. Nonetheless, the test should be tailored and the relevant parameters to assess should depend on the clinical indication.

The common parameters assessed during the ARM study are the following:

- *Resting pressure*:
    The resting pressure should be recorded only after the child is relaxed and comfortable. The basal resting sphincter pressure measurement with new technology of HRAM is simply obtained by inserting the catheter and evaluating in real-time the high-pressure zone over a period of 30 s [10]. Conversely, resting

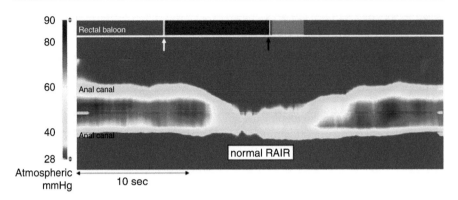

Fig. 8.1 Normal RAIR. *White* and *black arrows* point rectal balloon insufflation and deflation, respectively. The balloon inflation induces an increase in the rectal pressure, shown in the figure as *purple bar*. Normal RAIR is seen as a drop in anal canal pressure upon rectal balloon insufflation

pressure evaluation with low-resolution probes is usually performed through either stationary pull-through or continuous withdrawal [18]. The identification of high-pressure zone allows also the measurement of the anal canal length.

- *RAIR (recto-anal inhibitory reflex)* (Fig. 8.1):

    The RAIR consists in the relaxation of IAS upon a rectal distention. In pediatrics, there are no universally agreed criteria for its definition. It is currently defined as either a dropping in pressure by >5 mmHg or >15% of the resting pressure [18]. The drop in anal pressure may be difficult to be detected especially in uncooperative children and in patients with baseline low resting pressures (e.g., under anesthesia). The RAIR has a volume-dependent response: the larger the balloon volume, the greater the degree and duration of the relaxation. Its measurement is performed by rapidly inflating the rectal balloon with incremental volumes of 5 mL in infants and newborns (up to 20 mL) and increments of 10 mL in older children [10]. If complete relaxation is not obtained, volumes up to 250–300 mL can be reached in older children to elicit the RAIR. The absence of RAIR is suggestive of colonic aganglionosis or Hirschsprung disease (Fig. 8.2). The most common reason for a false-positive RAIR is represented by the migration of the probe during the procedure, which can be prevented by securing the catheter to the anal verge. Conversely, the most frequent cause for a false-negative RAIR test is rectal dilatation (i.e., megarectum), which does not allow the balloon to stretch the rectal walls (and therefore to generate the trigger pressure for the RAIR) because of the enlarged rectal volume [18].

- *Squeeze pressure* (Fig. 8.3):

    It is elicited by asking the child to voluntarily contract the anal canal and it is calculated as the greatest pressure increase referred to the baseline resting pressure. In some centers, the average of three measurements is calculated [10, 18]. An increased or decreased value may be due to myogenic or neurogenic causes.

- *Endurance squeeze* (Fig. 8.4):

    The child is asked to contract the anal canal as strongly as possible for at least 15- to 20-s period.

- *Rectal sensation*:

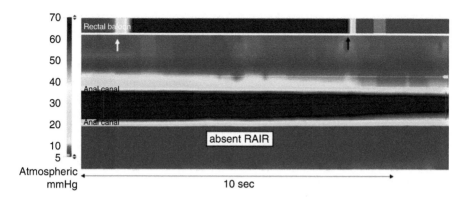

Fig. 8.2 Absent RAIR. *White* and *black arrows* point rectal balloon insufflation and deflation, respectively. The balloon inflation induces an increase in the rectal pressure, shown in the figure as *purple bar*. The anal sphincter pressure does not decrease upon rectal balloon insufflation. RAIR is absent in several conditions including colonic aganglionosis or Hirschsprung disease

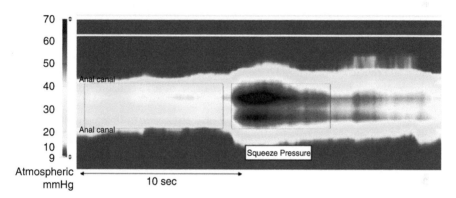

Fig. 8.3 Squeeze pressure. It is elicited by asking the child to voluntarily contract the anal sphincter. It is calculated as the greatest pressure increase referred to the baseline resting pressure

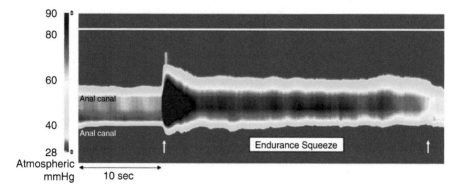

Fig. 8.4 Endurance squeeze. It is the length of time the child is able to maintain the anal canal pressure during a voluntary contraction. It is elicited by asking the child to voluntarily contract the anal sphincter as strongly as possible for a period of at least 15–20 s. The *white arrows* point the start and the end of the squeeze

The rectal sensation can be assessed in a cooperative child (usually aged 4–5 years and over) by steadily increasing the balloon size through the inflation of progressively greater volumes of water or air. It can be performed with or without deflation intervals in between the subsequent incremental volumes (intermittent rectal distension method or through ramp inflation method, respectively) [10]. It provides further information on the child's stool perception, which can be indicative of either anorectal dysfunction or dilated rectum. Three different sensation volumes are usually recorded: (i) *the first sensation*, which represents the lowest balloon volume at which the patient feels the balloon; (ii) *the urge sensation*, defined as the lowest volume required to elicit the defecation urge; (iii) *the maximum tolerable sensation*, reached when severe urgency and pain is experienced. This may be hard to be evaluated in children younger than 7 years of age and children with developmental impairment. Sensations are usually decreased in children with dilated rectum, often due to long-lasting outlet-obstruction constipation.

- *The bear-down maneuver or push (simulated defecation)* (Fig. 8.5):

  It is carried out to evaluate anorectal and pelvic floor pressure changes during a simulated defecation. Usually, this provocative test is possible to perform in children above 5–6 years of age and it requires significant cooperation. Normally, the defecation attempt should induce a simultaneous and coordinate increase in the rectal pressure and relaxation of anal sphincters. This maneuver allows clinicians to diagnose dyssynergic defecation, which is a common cause of fecal outlet obstruction.

- *Balloon expulsion test*:

  It is carried out asking the child to sit on a commode or in lateral position and expel the intrarectal inflated balloon, trying to guarantee as much privacy as possible. The test is defined normal if the balloon is expelled. In pediatrics, there is

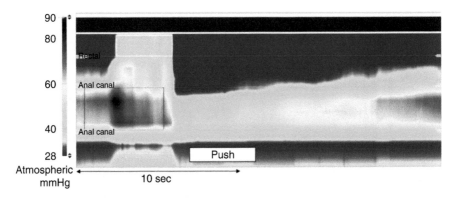

Fig. 8.5 Bear-down maneuver or push in dyssynergic defecation. It is carried out to evaluate anorectal and pelvic floor pressure changes during a simulated defecation. Normal defecation attempt induces a simultaneous and coordinate increase in the rectal pressure and relaxation of anal sphincters. In the figure, there is an increase in rectal pressure (*white square*) but paradoxical increase in anal pressure, consistent with the diagnose dyssynergic defecation, which is a common cause of fecal outlet obstruction in children

no a consensus on the time cut-off needed to expel the balloon and the ideal balloon volume. Studies have demonstrated that adult normal values can be used. Patients with dyssynergia usually fail to expel the balloon [19]. It has been demonstrated that this test in pediatric patients with outlet-obstruction type of constipation may help in tailoring therapeutic management [19].

8.3.3 Reference Values

In pediatric age, there is a lack of uniformity in terms of protocols and equipment, and hence lack of normal reference values. Moreover, normal HRAM and 3D HRAM values have been published only for adult populations [20–23], while only few studies have been performed in children with similar methodologies. Hence, the interpretation still relies on expertise of the pediatric gastroenterologists in the field. Moreover, conventional water-perfused ARM measures are routinely used in manometry reporting despite in adult literature has shown that the values with high-resolution manometry are higher than those with water perfusion [24]. Moreover, significant variability in values might depend on gender, BMI, age, use of different protocols, and the interaction between the patient and the clinician [21, 22, 25, 26].

To date only two studies in pediatric age have been performed using HARM and 3DHARM in order to establish normative values. One study using HARM reported normal values of anorectal sphincter metrics (including resting pressure, anal canal length, and RAIR) in 180 healthy and asymptomatic newborns based on age, and segregated by preterm vs term [27]. Recently, Banasiuk et al. have published a study aimed at evaluating normal 3DHRAM values in 61 children without symptoms from the lower gastrointestinal tract [8]. Normal values in pediatric age using either low- or high-resolution manometry are summarized in Tables 8.1 and 8.2.

Further studies are needed in pediatric populations in order to reach universally agreed normal values.

8.4 Indications

The indications of ARM are the following:

- *To rule out Hirschsprung disease (HD)*
  HD is characterized by the absence of ganglion cells in the myenteric and submucosal nerve plexuses in the colon and rectum secondary to an aberrant ontogenetic development of the gastrointestinal tract. Hence, due to the lack of innervation in the rectum, ARM shows a typical absence of IAS relaxation upon rectal distention. The absence of RAIR on ARM should prompt rectal suction biopsy (RSB), which is the gold standard for the diagnosis of HD. The absence of RAIR and the presence of ganglion cells at rectal suction biopsies define the condition named anal achalasia, which responds well to the treatment with botulin toxin [18].

Table 8.1 Normal manometric values in term and preterm neonates found in pediatric studies published using either low- or high-resolution anorectal manometry (Zar-Kessler et al. [18], modified)

	Equipment (technique)	Healthy patients (n)	Ages	Anal resting pressure (mmHg)	Anal canal length (cm)	RAIR threshold volume (mL)	Patients with normal RAIR (%)	Rectal pressure (mmHg)
Kumar et al. [2]	Water-perfused LR	30	3–28 D 34–39 weeks of GA	31.07 ± 10.9	1.67 ± 0.34	9.67 ± 3.7		
Benninga et al. [28]	Water-perfused LR	22	30–33 weeks PMA	32 ± 4		1.6 ± 0.3[a]	92%[a]	9 ± 2
			33–38 weeks PMA	51 ± 4		1.9 ± 0.2	100%	11 ± 3
de Lorijn et al. [29]	Water-perfused LR	16	3–23 D 27–30 weeks PMA	24.5 ± 11.4		3.4 ± 1.6[a]	81%[a]	6.5 ± 4.8
Tang et al. [27]	Water-perfused HRARM	85	0.5–85 D Preterm neonates 28–36 weeks of GA — ≤7 D	23.1 (19.9–26.2)	1.8 (1.7–2.0)	1.6 (1.4–1.9)		
			8–30 D	27.7 (24.8–30.6)	1.9 (1.7–2.0)	2.2 (1.7–2.7)		
			≥31 D[b]	32.9 (29.6–36.2)	2.0 (1.7–2.3)	3.7 (2.8–4.7)		
		95	1–67 D Term neonates 37–42 weeks of GA — ≤7 D	28.9 (25.8–32.0)	1.9 (1.7–2.1)	2.8 (2.3–3.3)		
			8–30 D	31.6 (28.9–34.3)	2.0 (1.9–2.1)	3.5 (2.9–4.0)		
			≥31 D[b]	39.9 (35.6–44.1)	2.3 (2.1–2.4)	4.5 (3.9–5.0)		

D days of life, LR low resolution, GA gestational age, PMA postmenstrual age
[a]Air insufflation: 1–5 mL of air was directly insufflated into the rectum to elicit the RAIR, instead of inflated balloon
[b]In this group healthy patients older than 1 month of life (infants) were included

Table 8.2 Normal manometric values for infants and children found in pediatric studies published using either low- or high-resolution anorectal manometry (Zar-Kessler et al. [18], modified)

	Equipment	Healthy patients (n)	Ages	Anal resting pressure (mmHg)	Anal canal length (cm)	Maximal squeeze pressure (mmHg)	RAIR threshold volume (mL)	First sensation volume (mL)	Critical volume (mL)	Rectal pressure (mmHg)
Benninga et al. [3]	Water-perfused LR	13	8–16 Y	55 ± 16		182 ± 61	18 ± 10	19 ± 12	131 ± 13	
Kumar et al. [2]	Water-perfused LR	30	35 D–16 M	42.43 ± 8.9	1.86 ± 0.6		14.0 ± 9.5			
Li et al. [30]	Not mentioned	30	18 M–12.3 Y	43.43 ± 8.79	3.03 ± 0.52		25.0 ± 11.6	28.0 ± 11.4	117.0 ± 46.2	
		10	7–14 Y		4.0 ± 0.9					
Sutphen et al. [31]	Water-perfused LR	27	6.5–12 Y[a]	80.9 ± 24.3		141.7 ± 47.2		30.4 ± 11.9	95.6 ± 38.1	13.0 ± 13.0 (resting) 60.5 ± 22.0 (defecation)
Banasiuk et al. [8]	Solid state 3DARM	9	2–5 Y	94 (24)	2.2 (0.5)	201 (60)[b]	13.3 (7.5)	34 (28.8)[c]	36 (27)[c]	
		19	5–8 Y	86 (15)	2.4 (0.4)	206 (40)[d]	11.1 (3.2)	25 (32.9)[d]	37.2 (35.9)[d]	
		19	9–12 Y	94 (15)	2.9 (0.6)	206 (59)	13.7 (5.9)	14.7 (6.9)	36.3 (19.8)	
		14	12–17 Y	96 (19)	3.1 (0.7)	229 (65)	18.6 (15.1)	22 (11.9)	55 (39.9)	

M months of age, *Y* years of age, *LR* low resolution

[a] Approximately

[b] Evaluated on seven patients

[c] Evaluated on five patients

[d] Evaluated on 18 patients

Recently, a new measure, the anal sphincter relaxation integral (ASRI), has been developed to objectively quantify the RAIR and discriminate patients with and without HD [32]. However, its role in the clinical management of patients with HD is still to be elucidated.

- *To evaluate the anorectal functions of HD children after surgical repair*

ARM plays an essential role in the post-surgical evaluation of these patients. For instance, it has been shown that the measurement of the length of the anal canal in HD children with fecal incontinence after surgical repair enables to pave further effective therapeutic management [33].

- *To evaluate the sphincter function in children with organic causes of constipation (e.g., anorectal malformation, spinal cord lesions)*

Children with anorectal malformations need an accurate functional evaluation after anorectal surgery in order to evaluate the residual anorectal function. Additionally, in the pre-surgery workup before reverting colostomy or ileostomy, ARM may be indicated in order to exclude the presence of outlet-obstruction defecation.

Spinal cord abnormalities may increase the tone of the anal sphincters as a consequence of the damage of upper motoneurons and an exaggerated contraction and anal spasms upon balloon dilation or sphincter relaxation with smaller balloon inflating volumes [34]. Conversely, in some neurological conditions the anal tone may be decreased due to abnormalities involving the lower motoneuron [35].

- *To evaluate persisting symptoms of constipation with or without fecal incontinence unresponsive to standard medical therapy*
- *To evaluate the anorectal function before and after therapeutic interventions such as botulinum toxin injection and biofeedback*
- *To assess the defecation dynamics*

The incoordination between the relaxation of the anal sphincters and pelvic floor muscles during defecation, called dyssynergic defecation, may be an underlying cause of constipation. This can be evaluated in real-time with ARM during the bear-down maneuver and, in adult population, ARM allows clinicians to differentiate dyssynergic defecation into different phenotypes according to the presence of adequate/inadequate increase in rectal pressure and failed reduction/paradoxical increase in anal pressure (type 1–4) [36]. Regardless of the type of ARM phenotype, dyssynergic defecation leads to outlet-obstruction constipation. This diagnosis can be confirmed by the inability of expelling the balloon. In children, both the bear-down maneuver and the balloon expulsion test may be falsely labelled as negative, because of the lateral position adopted during the test and the anxiety due to defecate in the presence of the clinicians [19].

8.5 Future Perspectives and Conclusions

Over the last decade, remarkable technical advances, in terms of probe miniaturization and pressure recording systems, have led to a more detailed understanding of the anorectal function. High-resolution (HRAM) and 3D high-definition

(3DHDAM) systems will gradually replace conventional low-resolution anorectal manometry. However, in children, although HRAM provides a greater characterization of defecatory disorders phenotypes, fecal incontinence, and anorectal dysmotility in adult population as well as in pediatric patients, it is still limited by the lack of standardization, interpretation, and normal data. The increasing application of new system in clinical will certainly lead to a substantial improvement of appropriate management driven by specific manometric patterns and underlying pathophysiological abnormalities.

References

1. Fritsch H, Brenner E, Lienemann A, Ludwikowski B. Anal sphincter complex: reinterpreted morphology and its clinical relevance. Dis Colon Rectum. 2002;45(2):188–94.
2. Kumar S, Ramadan S, Gupta V, Helmy S, Atta I, Alkholy A. Manometric tests of anorectal function in 90 healthy children: a clinical study from Kuwait. J Pediatr Surg. 2009;44(9):1786–90.
3. Benninga MA, Wijers OB, van der Hoeven CW, Taminiau JA, Klopper PJ, Tytgat GN, et al. Manometry, profilometry, and endosonography: normal physiology and anatomy of the anal canal in healthy children. J Pediatr Gastroenterol Nutr. 1994;18(1):68–77.
4. Bajwa A, Emmanuel A. The physiology of continence and evacuation. Best Pract Res Clin Gastroenterol. 2009;23(4):477–85.
5. Rasijeff AMP, Withers M, Burke JM, Jackson W, Scott SM. High-resolution anorectal manometry: a comparison of solid-state and water-perfused catheters. Neurogastroenterol Motil. 2017;29(11):13124. https://doi.org/10.1111/nmo.13124.
6. Lee TH, Bharucha AE. How to perform and interpret a high-resolution anorectal manometry test. J Neurogastroenterol Motil. 2016;22(1):46–59.
7. Ambartsumyan L, Rodriguez L, Morera C, Nurko S. Longitudinal and radial characteristics of intra-anal pressures in children using 3D high-definition anorectal manometry: new observations. Am J Gastroenterol. 2013;108(12):1918–28.
8. Banasiuk M, Banaszkiewicz A, Dziekiewicz M, Załęski A, Albrecht P. Values from three-dimensional high-resolution anorectal manometry analysis of children without lower gastrointestinal symptoms. Clin Gastroenterol Hepatol. 2016;14(7):993–1000.e3.
9. Di Lorenzo C, Hillemeier C, Hyman P, Loening-Baucke V, Nurko S, Rosenberg A, et al. Manometry studies in children: minimum standards for procedures. Neurogastroenterol Motil. 2002;14(4):411–20.
10. Rodriguez L, Sood M, Di Lorenzo C, Saps M. An ANMS-NASPGHAN consensus document on anorectal and colonic manometry in children. Neurogastroenterol Motil. 2017;29(1):12944. https://doi.org/10.1111/nmo.12944.
11. Tran K, Kuo B, Zibaitis A, Bhattacharya S, Cote C, Belkind-Gerson J. Effect of propofol on anal sphincter pressure during anorectal manometry. J Pediatr Gastroenterol Nutr. 2014;58(4):495–7.
12. Keshtgar AS, Choudhry MS, Kufeji D, Ward HC, Clayden GS. Anorectal manometry with and without ketamine for evaluation of defecation disorders in children. J Pediatr Surg. 2015;50(3):438–43.
13. Pfefferkorn MD, Croffie JM, Corkins MR, Gupta SK, Fitzgerald JF. Impact of sedation and anesthesia on the rectoanal inhibitory reflex in children. J Pediatr Gastroenterol Nutr. 2004;38(3):324–7.
14. Lamparyk K, Mahajan L, Debeljak A, Steffen R. Anxiety associated with high-resolution anorectal manometry in pediatric patients and parents. J Pediatr Gastroenterol Nutr. 2017;65(5):e98–e100.

15. Fortier MA, Kain ZN. Treating perioperative anxiety and pain in children: a tailored and innovative approach. Paediatr Anaesth. 2015;25(1):27–35.
16. Dias R, Baliarsing L, Barnwal NK, Mogal S, Gujjar P. Role of pre-operative multimedia video information in allaying anxiety related to spinal anaesthesia: a randomised controlled trial. Indian J Anaesth. 2016;60(11):843–7.
17. Lewis Claar R, Walker LS, Barnard JA. Children's knowledge, anticipatory anxiety, procedural distress, and recall of esophagogastroduodenoscopy. J Pediatr Gastroenterol Nutr. 2002;34(1):68–72.
18. Zar-Kessler C, Belkind-Gerson J. Anorectal manometry. In: NT CF, Di Lorenzo C, editors. Pediatric neurogastroenterology. Cham: Springer; 2017. p. 117–28.
19. Belkind-Gerson J, Goldstein AM, Kuo B. Balloon expulsion test as a screen for outlet obstruction in children with chronic constipation. J Pediatr Gastroenterol Nutr. 2013;56(1):23–6.
20. Carrington EV, Brokjaer A, Craven H, Zarate N, Horrocks EJ, Palit S, et al. Traditional measures of normal anal sphincter function using high-resolution anorectal manometry (HRAM) in 115 healthy volunteers. Neurogastroenterol Motil. 2014;26(5):625–35.
21. Noelting J, Ratuapli SK, Bharucha AE, Harvey DM, Ravi K, Zinsmeister AR. Normal values for high-resolution anorectal manometry in healthy women: effects of age and significance of rectoanal gradient. Am J Gastroenterol. 2012;107(10):1530–6.
22. Li Y, Yang X, Xu C, Zhang Y, Zhang X. Normal values and pressure morphology for three-dimensional high-resolution anorectal manometry of asymptomatic adults: a study in 110 subjects. Int J Color Dis. 2013;28(8):1161–8.
23. Coss-Adame E, Rao SS, Valestin J, Ali-Azamar A, Remes-Troche JM. Accuracy and Reproducibility of High-definition Anorectal Manometry and Pressure Topography Analyses in Healthy Subjects. Clin Gastroenterol Hepatol. 2015;13(6):1143–50.e1.
24. Vitton V, Ben Hadj Amor W, Baumstarck K, Grimaud JC, Bouvier M. Water-perfused manometry vs three-dimensional high-resolution manometry: a comparative study on a large patient population with anorectal disorders. Color Dis. 2013;15(12):e726–31.
25. Carrington EV, Grossi U, Knowles CH, Scott SM. Normal values for high-resolution anorectal manometry: a time for consensus and collaboration. Neurogastroenterol Motil. 2014;26(9):1356–7.
26. Lee HJ, Jung KW, Han S, Kim JW, Park SK, Yoon IJ, et al. Normal values for high-resolution anorectal manometry/topography in a healthy Korean population and the effects of gender and body mass index. Neurogastroenterol Motil. 2014;26(4):529–37.
27. Tang YF, Chen JG, An HJ, Jin P, Yang L, Dai ZF, et al. High-resolution anorectal manometry in newborns: normative values and diagnostic utility in Hirschsprung disease. Neurogastroenterol Motil. 2014;26(11):1565–72.
28. Benninga MA, Omari TI, Haslam RR, Barnett CP, Dent J, Davidson GP. Characterization of anorectal pressure and the anorectal inhibitory reflex in healthy preterm and term infants. J Pediatr. 2001;139(2):233–7.
29. de Lorijn F, Omari TI, Kok JH, Taminiau JA, Benninga MA. Maturation of the rectoanal inhibitory reflex in very premature infants. J Pediatr. 2003;143(5):630–3.
30. Li ZH, Dong M, Wang ZF. Functional constipation in children: investigation and management of anorectal motility. World J Pediatr. 2008;4(1):45–8.
31. Sutphen J, Borowitz S, Ling W, Cox DJ, Kovatchev B. Anorectal manometric examination in encopretic-constipated children. Dis Colon Rectum. 1997;40(9):1051–5.
32. Wu JF, Lu CH, Yang CH, Tsai IJ. Diagnostic role of anal sphincter relaxation integral in high-resolution anorectal manometry for Hirschsprung disease in infants. J Pediatr. 2018;194:136–41.e2.
33. Langer JC, Rollins MD, Levitt M, Gosain A, Torre L, Kapur RP, et al. Guidelines for the management of postoperative obstructive symptoms in children with Hirschsprung disease. Pediatr Surg Int. 2017;33(5):523–6.

34. Siddiqui A, Rosen R, Nurko S. Anorectal manometry may identify children with spinal cord lesions. J Pediatr Gastroenterol Nutr. 2011;53(5):507–11.
35. Huang YH. Neurogenic bowel: dysfunction and rehabilitation. In: Cifu DX, Lew HL, editors. Braddom's clinical handbook of physical medicine and rehabilitation. Amsterdam: Elsevier; 2018. p. 143–149.e7.
36. Ratuapli SK, Bharucha AE, Noelting J, Harvey DM, Zinsmeister AR. Phenotypic identification and classification of functional defecatory disorders using high-resolution anorectal manometry. Gastroenterology. 2013;144(2):314–22.e2.

Atlas

9

Sebastiano Bonventre, Gabriele Barletta, Salvatore Tolone, and Massimo Bellini

9.1 Resting Pressure

Resting pressure mainly results from the activity of the internal anal sphincter and is responsible for fecal continence at rest; it is also influenced by the hemorrhoidal plexus and the external anal sphincter pressure. Resting pressure is recorded after at least one minute of waiting (stabilization period) to allow the patient to adapt to the probe and to permit anal sphincter to stabilize at basal level.

Resting pressure recording, evaluated through an analysis of about 60 seconds with the patient at rest on his left side with the knees flexed, returns on the high resolution manometric color-contour plot an high pressure zone (HPZ), (Fig. 9.1, arrow 1), delimited by two low pressure zones (colder colors) proximally and distally representing, respectively, the rectum and the external environment.

On high definition 3D manometric image the resting pressure generates the so-called dumb-bell shape: this translates into a central high pressure ring reducing the caliber of the anal canal (arrow 2), with the yellow line indicating the anterior side of the anal canal (arrow 3) (Fig. 9.1).

During the analysis of resting pressure mean pressure, length of the HPZ and simmetry has to be evaluated.

S. Bonventre · G. Barletta (✉)
Department of Surgical, Oncological and Oral Sciences, Unit of General and Emergency Surgery, University of Palermo, Palermo, Italy

S. Tolone
Department of Medical, Surgical, Neurologic, Metabolic and Aging Sciences, General, Mininvasive and Obesity Surgery Unit, University of Campania "Luigi Vanvitelli", Naples, Italy

M. Bellini
Department of New Technologies and Translational Research in Medicine and Surgery, Gastroenterology Unit, University of Pisa, Pisa, Italy

© Springer Nature Switzerland AG 2020
M. Bellini (ed.), *High Resolution and High Definition Anorectal Manometry*,
https://doi.org/10.1007/978-3-030-32419-3_9

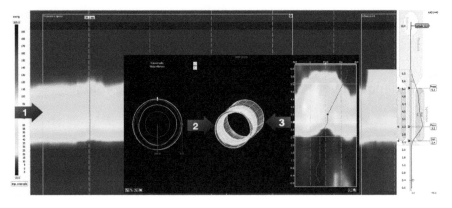

Fig. 9.1 Resting pressure

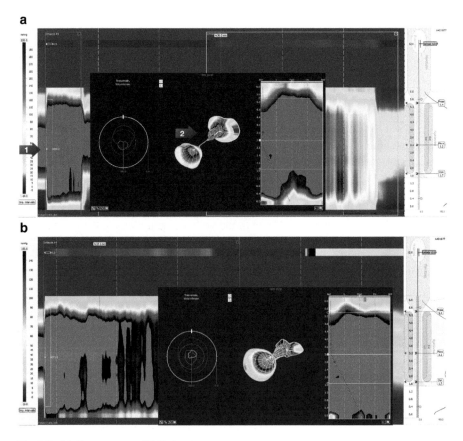

Fig. 9.2 (**a**) Short squeeze, (**b**) Endurance squeeze

PUSH

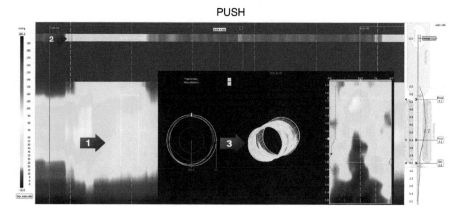

Fig. 9.3   Push

9.2   Squeeze

The contractile activity of the external anal sphincter muscle is evaluated by asking the patient to perform three consecutive maximal anal contractions of 5 seconds each (short squeeze, Fig. 9.2a) and one 30 seconds long squeeze (endurance squeeze, Fig. 9.2b).

The voluntary contraction maneuver causes a pressure increase on the high resolution manometric color-contour plot with warm colors appearence (in Fig. 9.2, peak pressure 356.0 mmHg, arrow 1).

On 3D high definition image the squeezing maneuver generates an hourglass shape appearance (Fig. 9.2, arrow 2): it is possible to appreciate a central pressure peak that causes the total or sub-total obliteration of the anal canal, bounded by two low pressure zones, proximally and distally.

The 3D image also allows to detect asymmetry of the external anal sphincter contraction (for example, asymmetry due to traumatic or iatrogenic damage), otherwise not detectable through simple 2D high resolution evaluation.

9.3   Push

In physiological conditions, the pushing maneuver leads to an increase of the abdominal pressure (as a consequence of the bearing down maneuver) associated with anal canal relaxation. The simulated defecation is repeated at least three times with the patient lying on his left side.

On the high resolution color-contour, it is possible to appreciate a shift towards colder colors (Fig. 9.3, arrow 1) on the sphincter apparatus corresponding to physiological sphincterial relaxation (in Fig. 9.3, relaxing pressure: 37.4 mmHg); on the rectal sensor color-contour (arrow 2), it is necessary to verify the effective pressure increase testifying that an adequate bearing down maneuver is performed by the patient: rectal pressure increase is efficient when it exceeds at least 40 mmHg.

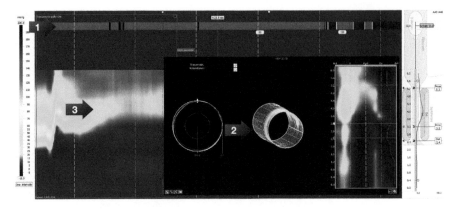

Fig. 9.4 Recto-anal inhibitory reflex

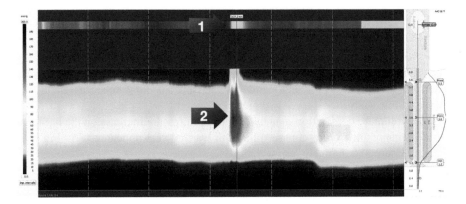

Fig. 9.5 Cough reflex

On the 3D high definition manometric image the simulated defecation generates a symmetric increase in the caliber of the functional anal canal (arrow 3) compared to the seconds immediately preceding the pushing maneuver.

9.4   Recto-Anal Inhibitory Reflex

The evaluation of the recto-anal inhibitory reflex (RAIR) involves the distension of the rectum walls through the progressive insufflation of air inside the balloon placed on the anorectal manometry probe.

The pressure increase appreciated in the rectum (arrow 1), if reflex arc is preserved, will correspond to a relaxation of the sphincterial apparatus which, in the 3D manometric image, results in an increase in the caliber of the functional anal canal (arrow 2) compared to the seconds immediately preceding the air blowing. On the 2D manometric color-contour plot a color change towards the colder colors (arrow 3) of the pressure scale is shown RAIR may be elicited by 20 ml air blowing, but is

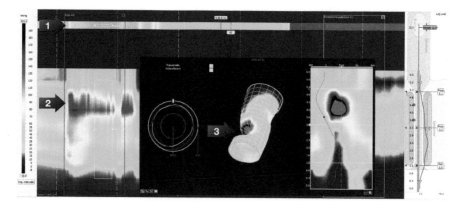

Fig. 9.6 Paradoxical puborectalis contraction

good practice to evaluate it with progressive insufflations until reaching a value of at least 60 ml.

9.5 Cough Reflex

The evaluation of the cough reflex allows to verify the integrity of the reflex arc. It is composed of the pudendal nerves and sacral roots, which permits fecal continence during such maneuvers: the act of cough causes an increase in intraabdominal pressure to which corresponds a rise in sphincter pressure caused by external sphincter muscle contraction. Loss of this reflex, due to neurological or mechanical causes, such as traumas or nerve compression, could lead to episodes of fecal incontinence.

In Fig. 9.5 it is possible to notice, during cough maneuver, a pressure rising in the rectal sensors (arrow 1) which activates the physiological reflex arc that causes contraction of the external sphincter muscle (warmer colors along sphincter sensors) (arrow 2).

9.6 Paradoxical Puborectalis Contraction

The paradoxical puborectalis contraction is a dyssynergic condition of the pelvic floor muscles that may appear during straining: in physiological conditions the puborectalis muscle sling, during wilting, undergoes a relaxation, straightening the way of expulsion of the stools.

In this type of dyssynergic defecation there is a muscular incoordination characterized by a paradoxical contraction of the puborectalis muscle. In this patients a correct propulsive thrust through the bearing down maneuver is detectable (Fig. 9.6, arrow 1) but the paradoxical contraction of the pubo-rectal is sling prevents physiological evacuation, leading to an obstructed defecation.

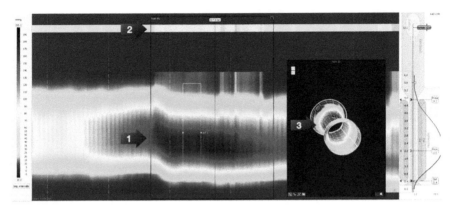

Fig. 9.7 Paradoxical contraction with external anal sphincter recruitment

This dyssynergic condition manifests itself on the high resolution manometric color-contour plot, while patient is asked to strain, with a pressure change towards warmer colors (rather than the physiological color change towards colder colors) with its peak on the proximal portion of the functional anal canal (arrow 2) (Fig. 9.6).

High definition manometric image allows to appreciate the presence of an asymmetrical pressure increase located on the posterior portion of the anal canal (arrow 3), due to the typical sling course of the puborectalis muscle.

9.7 Paradoxical Contraction with External Anal Sphincter Recruitment

Paradoxical contraction during straining with external anal sphincter recruitment is shown in Fig. 9.7: the 2D manometric color plot shows a change towards warmer colors represented all along the anal sphincter (arrow 1) due to paradoxical contraction of the external anal sphincter, associated with rectal pressure increase (arrow 2) due to bearing down maneuver.

3D high definition manometric image shows a diffuse caliber reduction of the anal canal (arrow 3): it is noteworthy that in this patient it is not possible to appreciate the posterior pressure increase typical of paradoxical puborectalis contraction.

9.8 Anal Sphincter Impaired Relaxation

The anal sphincter impaired relaxation is also a dyssynergic phenomenon that manifests itself during simulated defecation: on the 2D manometric color-contour plot it is possible to appreciate a correct propulsive thrust during the bearing down maneuver (Fig. 9.8, arrow 1) associated, in this case, with an absence of the color change

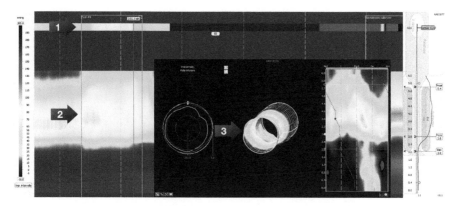

Fig. 9.8 Anal sphincter impaired relaxation

towards the colder colors of the pressure scale (as one would expect to find in case of physiological conditions); anal sphincter impaired relaxation is characterized, instead, by a permanence of the high pressure zone (arrow 2) compared to the pre-pushing phase.

The physiological increase in the caliber of the anal canal is not appreciated in the 3D high definition manometric image; on the contrary, it is possible to detect the constant presence of the "dumb-bell shape" image appreciable in resting condition (arrow 3).

9.9 Insufficient Resting Pressure

An impaired resting pressure could lead to episodes of fecal incontinence: the major predisposing factor is certainly childbirth and possible peripartum episiotomy; other causes can be traumatic sphincter lesions, neurological causes, inflammatory bowel diseases, or iatrogenic causes secondary to surgery for anal fissures, perianal fistulas, or tumors.

In Fig. 9.9a it is possible to appreciate a reduced resting pressure: the HPZ is characterized by reduced length and colder colors of the manometric scale (arrow 1) if compared to physiological pattern. The 3D high definition image shows an increased caliber of the anal canal at rest (arrow 2) compared to physiological dumbbell appearence.

Figure 9.9b shows the correspondent conventional manometry pattern: mean resting pressure value is 30.4 mmHg, with a pressure peak of 33.2 mmHg.

In Fig. 9.10 a complete abolition of the resting pressure is showed in a patient affected by ulcerative colitis and stoma carrier; 2D manometric colour plot shows that no pressure is detected (arrow 2); the 3D manometric image shows a marked increase in the caliber of the anal canal (arrow 1), with complete disappearance of the handlebar image that characterizes physiological resting pressure.

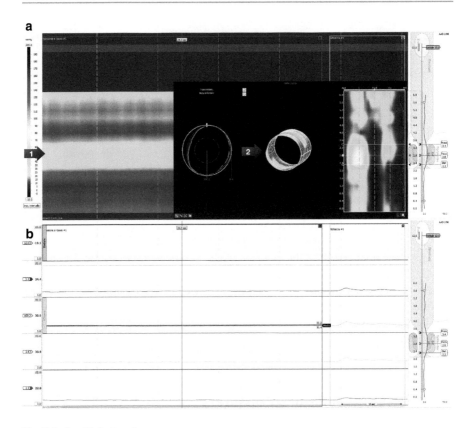

Fig. 9.9 Insufficient resting pressure

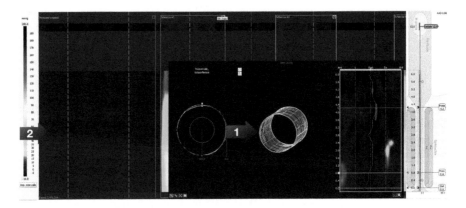

Fig. 9.10 Resting pressure abolition in patient affected by ulcerative colitis and stoma carrier

9.10 Insufficient Squeezing

The physiological contraction of the external anal sphincter generates on the 2D high resolution color-contour a color change towards warmer colors maintained over time and, at the 3D high definition image, a reduction in the size of the functional anal canal.

In Fig. 9.11 an insufficient voluntary contraction is shown in a patient affected by multiple sclerosis: during squeezing the high pressure zone does not reach the warmer colors of the pressure scale as one would expect in physiological conditions, not even on his peak pressure (maximum contraction: 101.0 mmHg, arrow 2).

The 3D manometric image shows how, during contraction, the anal canal does not completely close, but it remains widely open instead (arrow 1), although without any signs of asymmetry.

9.11 Anal Sphincter Lesion

A sphincter lesion can be the consequence of different events: causes could be rapresented by vaginal delivery with consequent obstetric implications but it can be also caused by traumas or iatrogenic causes.

It can cause active fecal incontinence, with urgency and persistence of the evacuation stimulus, but it can also provoke fecal soiling.

In Fig. 9.12 a iatrogenic lesion of the external anal sphincter muscle in a patient who underwent sphincterotomy for a trans-sphincteric fistula.

Through high resolution anorectal manometry the consequences of external anal sphincter lesion can be appreciable during voluntary contraction: on the 2D manometric color plot it is possible to appreciate a pressure increase with a change towards the warmer colors (arrow 2) which may not reach the highers colors of the manometric scale and appear insufficient, but without providing any information on the possible site of the injury.

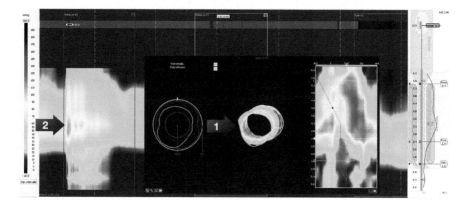

Fig. 9.11 Insufficient squeezing

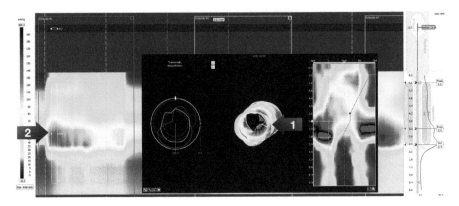

Fig. 9.12 External anal sphincter lesion

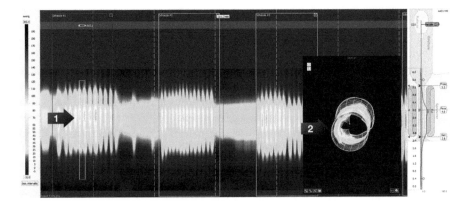

Fig. 9.13 Anal sphincter traumatic damage

On the contrary, 3D high definition evaluation is particularly useful in this context since, during voluntary contraction, it is possible to appreciate a marked asymmetry of the high pressure zone (arrow 1) otherwise not detectable through simple high resolution evaluation. External anal sphincter activity is maintained in this patient only along the anterior side of the anal canal, and it is reduced along the posterior side.

In Fig. 9.13 the manometric features of a traumatic damage of external anal sphincter muscle are shown: the 2D manometric color-contour shows multiple pressure peaks (warmer colors, arrow 1) characterized by short duration and insufficient strength (pressure displayed: 81.3 mmHg); 3D manometric image highlights an asymmetrical contraction characterized by muscular activity represented only along the posterior side of the anal canal (arrow 2).

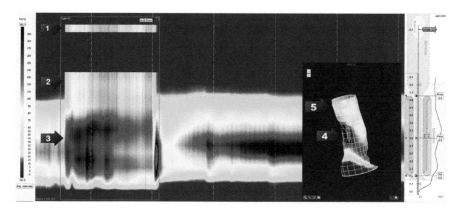

Fig. 9.14 Puborectalis paradoxical contraction in patient affected by rectal prolapse

9.12 Rectal Prolapse

During high resolution and high definition manometric study it could be possible to appreciate rectal prolapse in straining phase: in Fig. 9.14 it is possible to notice how in the 2D high resolution manometric color plot, during an adequate bearing down maneuver, pressure increase occours not only in the rectal sensor (arrow 1), but warmer colors also appears to descend into anal canal (arrow 2). The color plot shows also how in the anal canal pressure increase is compatible with dyssynergic defecation (arrow 3) (Fig. 9.14).

On 3D manometric image, it is shown the puborectalis asymmetrical pressure increase (arrow 4) associated with a proximal caliber reduction of the anal canal during simulated defecation (arrow 5).

In Fig. 9.15, a rectal prolapse in patient who underwent STARR is reported: arrow 1 shows a pressure increase above the anal sphincter during bearing down maneuver; arrow 2 shows the conventional manometry trace with a diffuse pressure increase during such maneuver.

In Fig. 9.16 physiological anal sphincter relaxation in patient affected by rectal prolapse is reported: during simulated defecation pressure increase occurs not only in the rectal sensor (due to bearing down maneuver), but warmer colors seems to descend also above the anal sphincter (arrow 1), descending even more on successive bearing down maneuver (arrow 2). This aspect occurs however in presence of a sufficient relaxation of the anal sphincter: the 2D manometric color plot shows, in correspondence with the correct bearing down maneuver, a color change towards colder colors along the anal sphincter (arrow 3) (Fig. 9.16).

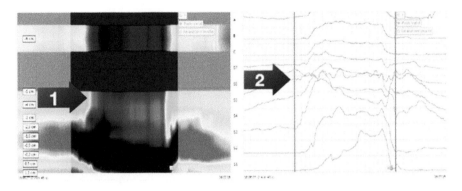

Fig. 9.15 Rectal prolapse recurrence after STARR

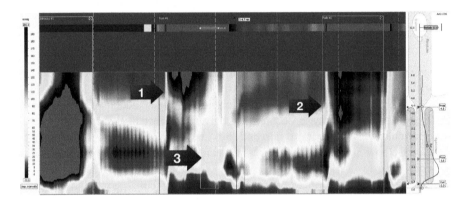

Fig. 9.16 Physiological anal sphincter relaxation in patient affected by rectal prolapse

9.13   Anal Fissure

Patients suffering from anal fissure may present an internal sphincter hypertonia which can slow down or prevent the resolution of the ulceration.

In Fig. 9.17 altered resting pressure in patient affected by anal fissure is shown: high resolution manometric color-contour plot shows a high pressure zone characterized by warmer colors (arrow 1) if compared to physiological conditions during resting pressure recording. The 3D high definition image is characterized by symmetrical caliber reduction of the anal canal (arrow 2) if compared to physiological dumb-bell shape appearence.

9.14 Neurologic Damage in Previous Cerebral Hemorrhage Due to Vascular Malformation

In Fig. 9.18 an impaired perineum due to cerebral hemorrhage secondary to vascular malformation: it is easily noticed how every step of the manometric study does not elicit any response along the sphincterial apparatus: during cough, in physiological conditions, a contraction of the external anal sphincter is expected, contrary to what happens in this patient, in which no response is appreciated during such a maneuver (arrow 1); also during voluntary contraction and simulated defecation (arrows 2 and 3, respectively), no activity is recorded along the sphincterial sensors, with permanence of the HPZ.

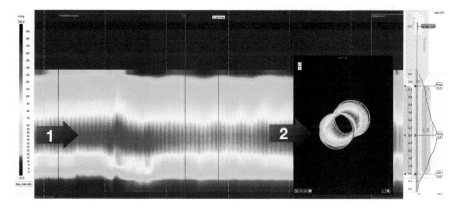

Fig. 9.17 Anal fissure

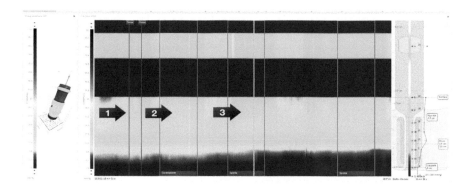

Fig. 9.18 Neurologic damage in previous cerebral hemorrhage

9.15 Hirschsprung's Disease

In Fig. 9.19 a case of Hirschsprung disease diagnosed in childhood is reported: the air insufflation in the balloon, with consequent pressure increase on the rectal sensor (arrow 1), does not correspond to the physiological relaxation of the sphincterial apparatus; on the contrary, the permanence of the high pressure zone (arrow 2) is appreciable.

In Fig. 9.20, even after ten balloon filling maneuvers (maximum air insufflations 240 cc) (arrow 1), no rectal-anal inhibitory reflex is appreciated on the sphincterial sensors, with permanence of the HPZ on the high resolution manometric color-contour (arrow 2) and reduced caliber on the 3D high definition reconstruction (arrow 3).

RAIR

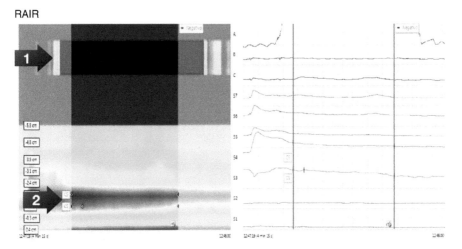

Fig. 9.19 Hirschprung disease

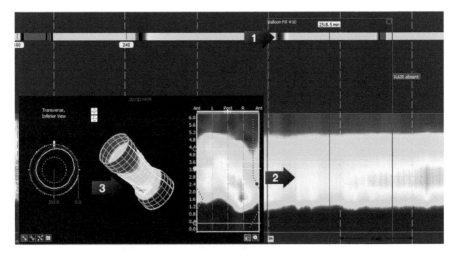

Fig. 9.20 Rectal-anal inhibitory reflex absence after multiple balloon insufflation

9.16   Push Maneuver in Patient with Uterine Pessary

In Fig. 9.21 simulated defecation maneuver in a female patient with uterine pessary for uterine prolapse is shown. During adequate bearing down maneuver, an accessory high pressure zone descending along the sphincterial sensors (arrow 1) is detectable. Unlike the color-contour plot that characterizes patients suffering from rectal prolapse, in this patient warmer colors are not diffuse over the sphincterial apparatus, but are defined by a short pressure area descending towards the anal canal.

On the 3D image pressure is detected only along the anterior sensors of the high definition manometric probe (arrow 2); this is compatible with the anatomical position of the uterine pessary.

9.17   Dyssynergic Defecation Classification According to Rao

Type I dyssynergic defecation is characterized by an adequate bearing down maneuver that generates an increase in rectal pressure equal or greater than 40 mmHg (arrows 1) associated with paradoxical puborectalis contraction: arrow 2 shows the pressure increase along the anal canal during bearing down maneuver (Fig. 9.22).

In type II dyssynergic defecation, during bearing down maneuver, an insufficient propulsive force along the rectal canal is generated (arrow 1 shows no pressure increase in the rectal sensor) associated with paradoxical increase in anal sphincter pressure (arrows 2) (Fig. 9.23).

Type III dyssynergic defecation is characterized by an adequate rectal pressure increase (arrow 1 shows a pressure increase greater than 40 mmHg) during bearing

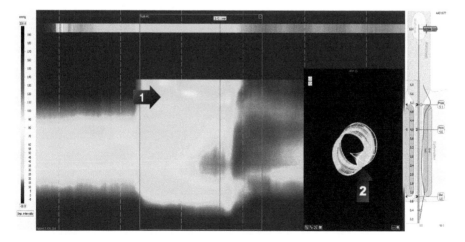

Fig. 9.21 Push maneuver in patient with uterine pessary

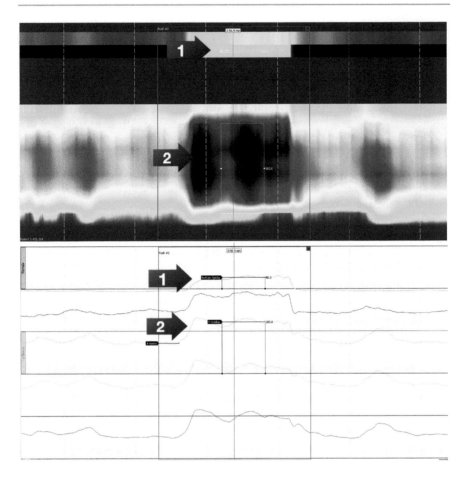

Fig. 9.22 Type I

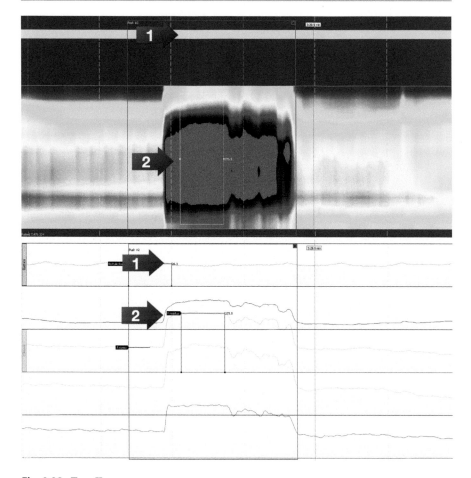

Fig. 9.23 Type II

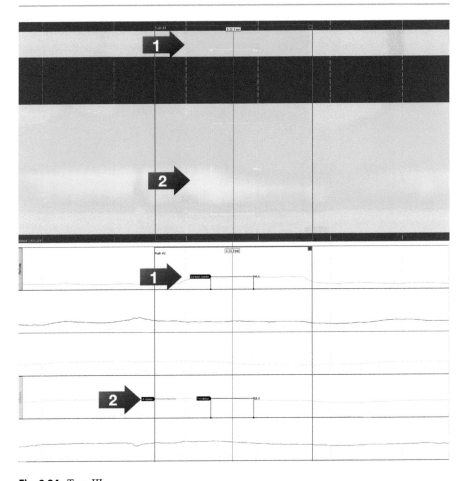

Fig. 9.24 Type III

down maneuver associated with absent or insufficient anal sphincter relaxation (pressure reduction equal or less than 20%) (arrow 2) (Fig. 9.24).

In type IV dyssynergic defecation the subject is unable to generate an adequate propulsive force during bearing down maneuver (arrow 1 shows an insufficient pressure increase in the rectal sensor) associated with absent or insufficient anal sphincter relaxation (arrow 2) (Fig. 9.25).

9.18   Artifacts

Artifacts may be due to probe calibration errors or damage of certain sensors.

In Fig. 9.26a high definition manometric color plot shows different high pressure zones with low pressure areas between them (arrows 1): this image could generate the suspect of an altered anatomy of the anal canal. On the 3D

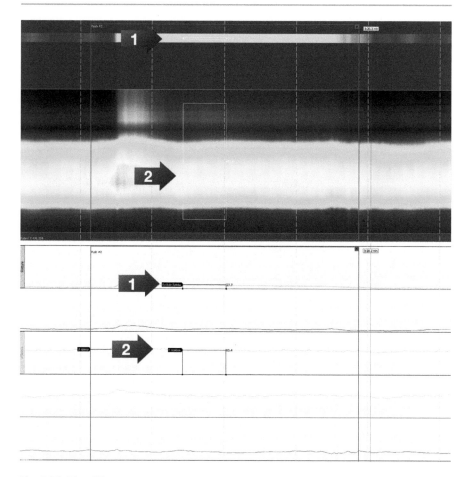

Fig. 9.25 Type IV

manometric image, it is possible to notice that the anal canal reconstruction seems to be also remarkably altered.

The artifact reason can be easily noticed in Fig. 9.26b, in which, after removing the probe (arrow 2) it continues to record multiple high and low pressure areas associated with an altered 3D reconstruction: when no pressure is applied on the manometric sensors, a diffuse low pressure plot should be expected.

This particular artifact can be generated by a damaged probe sensor or by errors during the application of the protective sheath.

In Fig. 9.27 artifact is due to the dislocation of the elastic device that keeps the balloon in place: it is possible to notice a high pressure zone (warmer colors, arrow 1) appearing in the rectal sensor and how it does not disappear even after balloon air removal or after probe movements.

The dislocation of the elastic device on the rectal sensor is responsible for the high pressure zone reported.

ARTIFACTS

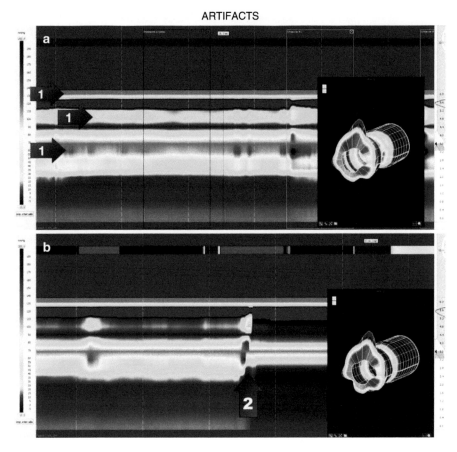

Fig. 9.26 Probe calibration error

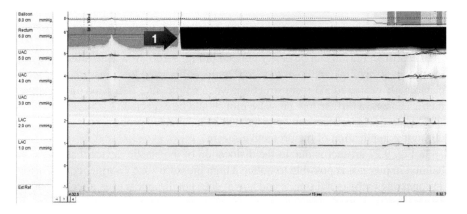

Fig. 9.27 Balloon and elastic device dislocation

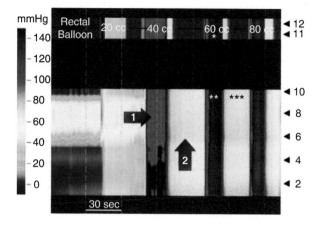

Fig. 9.28 Air trapping

Fig. 9.28 shows an artifact generated by air trapped in the probe protective sheath: a loose tie between the balloon, positioned at the top of the probe, and the sheath can lead to an air escape from the balloon to the protective sheath, generating a pressure increase, detected by the sphincterial sensors, during (arrow 1) and between (arrow 2) successive air insufflation maneuvers (*reproduced with permission from Conklin et al.* [1]).

Reference

1. Conklin J, Pimentel M, Soffer E. (2009) Color Atlas of High Resolution Manometry. https://doi.org/10.1007/978-0-387-88295-6.

Renato Bocchini, Michela Zari, Pasquale Talento, and Andrea Pancetti

Anal resting pressure: Pressure detectable at rest in static conditions. Baseline anal pressure profiles show a peak pressure in the range of 70–80 mmHg at a level of 1.6 cm from the anal verge, which corresponds to the level of the IAS. In addition, there is a hump in the posterior pressure from 2.4 cm to 4 cm corresponding to the puborectalis muscle. Pressures are markedly asymmetric in the axial and circumferential directions. *Mean resting (MeRAP) and maximal resting anal pressure (MRAP)* are measured by the software in the highest pressure zone of the anal canal. Resting pressure is the pressure in the high-pressure zone at rest after a period of stabilization. Maximum resting pressure is the highest resting pressure recorded [1–4].

Anal sphincter relaxation integral (ASRI): it has been developed mimicking the distal contractile integral determined by HR esophageal manometry to calculate the integral of contractile amplitude × duration × length (mmHg-s-cm of the distal esophageal contraction exceeding 20 mmHg from the transition zone to the proximal margin of the lower esophageal sphincter); it is used to quantify the RAIR; ASRI <10, 15, and 20 mmHg (ASRI10, ASRI15, and ASRI20, respectively) in an observed time window is used to quantify the amplitude of RAIR [5].

Balloon expulsion test (BET): the ability to evacuate is tested by BET: patients are asked to expel a 50 mL water-filled balloon attached to a Foley catheter sitting on a commode in privacy. According to the most authors the test has to be stopped if the balloon is not expelled within 2 or 3 min. A balloon expulsion time (BET) <120/180 s is considered normal. If patient could not expel the balloon

R. Bocchini (✉)
GI Unit, Physiopathology Lab, Malatesta Novello Private Hospital, Cesena, Italy

M. Zari · A. Pancetti
Gastrointestinal Unit, Department of Translational Research and New Technologies in Medicine and Surgery, University of Pisa, Pisa, Italy

P. Talento
Department of General Surgery, U.O.C. Nord Area - AUSL IRCCS, Reggio Emilia, Italy

© Springer Nature Switzerland AG 2020
M. Bellini (ed.), *High Resolution and High Definition Anorectal Manometry*,
https://doi.org/10.1007/978-3-030-32419-3_10

spontaneously, the balloon can be connected over a pulley to external weights, starting with 50 g and increasing, up to a maximum of 564 g [6–9].

Cough reflex test: the evaluation of anal and rectal pressures (the difference between the maximum pressure recorded during a voluntary cough and the resting pressure at the same level in the anal canal) is important in the evaluation of fecal incontinence; indeed, the ability of increasing the anal canal pressures during abrupt rise in intra-abdominal pressure is an important mechanism in maintaining continence. This maneuver evaluates the integrity of spinal reflex pathways in patients with fecal incontinence. The patient is asked to cough or inflate a balloon. Normally, the increased abdominal pressure triggers the external anal sphincter contraction. The maneuver can be repeated more than once [10].

Defecation index (or rectoanal index): it is a ratio of the intra-rectal pressure and anal sphincter residual pressure [11, 12]. During normal defecation, it is intuitive that rectal pressure should exceed anal pressure. The defecation index is a simple and useful quantitative assessment of rectoanal co-ordination during defecation. A normal defecation index is >1.5. An index <1.3 has been used to diagnose dyssynergia with non-HRM. However, several studies have observed that approximately 20% of asymptomatic people have dyssynergic defecation during HRM.

Dumb-bell: with 3-D maps, the resting frame shows a dumb-bell shape, with a high-pressure ring in the middle and low-pressure areas on both ends [10].

Dyssynergia: it is characterized by a paradoxical contraction of anal sphincter and\or puborectalis muscle during the bear-down maneuvers, or by failure of these muscles to appropriately relax during attempted defecation [13].

Functional anal canal length: it is defined as the area over which the resting anal pressures exceed the resting intrarectal pressure by at least 5 mmHg [10].

Functional defecation disorders: dyssynergia can be additionally categorized, according to Rome IV criteria [14], into four types on anorectal manometry data, based on patient ability to generate adequate pushing force and the type of sphincter contraction:

1. Type I dyssynergia is characterized by adequate rectal propulsion with paradoxical anal contraction.
2. Type II dyssynergia is characterized by impaired rectal propulsion associated with paradoxical anal contraction.
3. Type III dyssynergia is characterized by adequate rectal propulsion with an incomplete anal relaxation.
4. Type IV dyssynergia is characterized by impaired rectal propulsion with incomplete anal relaxation.

HDAM or 3-D high-definition anorectal pressure manometry/topography: only HDAM provides the pressures measured by individual sensors around the catheter circumference and is able to three-dimensionally reconstruct the anorectum by color and morphology of anal canal, based on pressure changes detected by 256 circumferential sensors (compared to the 12 sensors on the standard 2D HRAM catheter), providing a more global assessment of function [4, 15, 16].

HPZ (high-pressure zone): it is defined as the length of the anal canal with a resting pressure at least 30% higher than rectal pressure [1]. This is automatically determined by the software. The Sierra HRM system calculates HPZ as the length of the average pressure profile in the resting pressure frame defined as {rectal pressure + [(anal resting pressure − rectal pressure) × 0.25].

HRAM (high-resolution anorectal manometry): it utilizes flexible catheters (water perfused or solid state catheters) that typically house longitudinal sensors spaced approximately 0.6–1 cm apart. The most proximal one or two sensors (often spaced further apart) may be used to record intra balloon pressure within a balloon attached to the uppermost part of the catheter for rectal distension/sensory testing [4, 15].

Both for HDAM and HRAM, there are currently two systems in practice: those that use solid state probes (the 3-D high-resolution solid probe has 256 pressure sensors on 16 lines, with each line having 16 circumferential sensors; the probe has a diameter of 10.75 mm, a length of 64 mm, an internal lumen to inflate the balloon −3.3 cm long with a capacity of 400 cm—and needs a disposable sheath) and those with continuous water perfusion (using a 24-channel anorectal manometry probe) [17]. Internal anal sphincter, external anal sphincter, and puborectalis function and integrity can be assessed at rest, during attempted squeeze maneuvers and during strain (bear-down) maneuver; a manometric investigation comprises a number of separate tests, with the selection (and order) of test maneuvers performed conforming issues, symptoms and reason for referral. Test components may include assessment of anal canal length; anal resting tone; anal squeeze pressure; the recto-anal inhibitory reflex; recto-anal (pressure) co-ordination on coughing; recto-anal (pressure) co-ordination during the "push" maneuver; rectal sensations and the evaluation of the relationship between inflated volume and rectal pressure, often improperly defined as "compliance".

Integrated pressurized volume (IPV): it's a measure of anal relaxation during simulated evacuation. The IPV not only reflects the anal pressure (amplitude), but also the duration of relaxation and the spatial component (i.e. length of anal canal) [18]. It is calculated by multiplying amplitude, distance and time. This new parameter makes more precise measurement of muscular contractility in the anal canal. Moreover, it has been reported that IPV was more strongly correlated with BET time in asymptomatic individuals than the previously used conventional parameters [19].

Isobaric contour: it is the line which identifies the loci in the anorectal pressure topography where the pressure is at the same level.

Maximum voluntary pressure: it is the highest pressure recorded above the baseline (0) at any level of the anal canal during maximum squeeze effort performed by the patient.

Push or straining (simulated evacuation without rectal distention): to assess defecation dynamics, patient is asked to attempt defecation by pushing three times

(1 min apart), *bearing down* (*straining to defecate*) as if he was "on-commode or toilet.". This maneuver allows to measure pressure during attempted defecation, or so-called simulated defecation. An increase in intrarectal pressures (due to the Valsalva maneuver with abdominal muscles contraction) and the drop of pressures in the anal canal are reported in normal subjects. The HDAM image of the bear-down maneuver shows the change of resting pressures (of cylindrical shape) to *trumpet s*hape as a result of increased intrarectal pressures and reduced anal pressures [10].

Rectal compliance: it is measured from the data obtained during intermittent intrarectal balloon insufflations. Balloon distension causes an initial increase in the intra balloon (rectal) pressure which is followed by a gradual decline in pressure to a steady state value (as the rectum accommodates to the increased volume). Compliance is then calculated as change in balloon volume divided by change in intra balloon pressure. Increased compliance can be related to the presence of mega-rectum. Decreased compliance is related to reduced rectal adaptability, as in procti-tis (both inflammatory and actinic), "sphincter saving operations," etc.; reduced elasticity compromises tonic rectal adaptability and can cause rectal fasic contrac-tion (possible cause of incontinence). The rectal balloons supplied with some mano-metric catheters are relatively stiff. These balloons can be cleaned and reused, so the balloons stiffness varies over time. For this reason, rectal compliance and pressure thresholds for rectal sensations cannot be reliably measured with anorectal manom-etry; rectal compliance should be assessed using the barostat (provided with a long infinitely compliant polyethylene bag) [20].

Rectal sensitivity: it is evaluated by measuring the perception of rectal distention performed by placing a balloon catheter above the anorectal ring; *rectal sensitivity testing* involves progressive filling of the rectal balloon with an increasing volume of air or liquid. The volume at which the patient can perceive the presence of the inflated balloon (minimum rectal volume perceived by the patient)—is the *first sen-sation*. During further gradual inflation the volume at which the patient reports *the desire to defecate (constant sensation)* and the volume at which the patient experi-ences elevated discomfort and an intense desire to defecate *(maximum tolerated volume)* are recorded. The threshold can vary according to the different methods of inflation (continuous or intermittent) and to the shape and the material of the bal-loon [2, 3].

Rectoanal inhibitory reflex (RAIR): it is an anal reflex response, described mano-metrically by the relaxation pressure or loss of anal canal pressure during rectal balloon distention [21]. The relaxation pressure is a function of rectal distention volume. The relaxation pressure is also dependent on the recording location along the anal canal. Adequate RAIR is defined as transient decrease in resting anal pres-sure by >50% of basal pressure in response to rapid inflation of a rectal balloon.

Rectoanal pressure gradient (RAPG): it is an integrated function of rectal pres-surization and sphincter relaxation/opening during 'simulated defecation [4, 15, 22] and is calculated as the pressure difference between rectal and anal pressures taken over 2 s at the highest rectoanal pressure gradient during pushing period.

Percentage of anal relaxation is taken according to (1-residual anal pressure/anal resting pressure) × 100 where residual anal pressure is taken over 2 s.

Sand clock: the "sand clock" appearance on 3-D or the "λ" shape on 2-D mapping during the squeezing maneuver is typical of a normal function of the external anal sphincter muscle [10].

Sensory-motor response: it is a transient anal contraction following the rectoanal inhibitory reflex.

Sleeve sensor or *electronic sleeve*: it obtains stable measurements of sphincter pressure by recording the maximum pressure between two markers placed above and below the high-pressure zone at the anal sphincter. The eSleeve option in the software reduces pressures recorded across the longitudinal extent of the anal canal into a single value, at rest, during squeeze, and during rectal distention. It identifies the highest of all pressures recorded by anal sensors at every point in time and is used to calculate the average and maximum anal resting pressure and the maximum squeeze pressure. During simulated evacuation, the eSleeve identifies the most positive (or least negative) difference (i.e., rectoanal gradient) between rectal and anal (rectal–anal) pressure over a 20-s period. HRAM measurements of anal sphincter pressures at rest and during squeeze are higher than the corresponding pressures recorded with conventional manometry because of the eSleeve function, which uses the highest pressures recorded at any level of the anal canal at every instant in time [4].

Sphincter endurance: it is the length of time that the patient can maintain a squeeze pressure above the resting pressure [2].

Squeeze pressure: it is the pressure increment above resting pressure after voluntary squeeze contraction and is a calculated value that is the difference between the maximum voluntary pressure and the resting pressure at the same level of the anal canal [10]. Squeeze pressures are greater in the lower anterior part of anal canal, as compared to the remaining part of anal canal ($p = 0.017$). Altered sphincteric voluntary contraction is connected to external anal sphincter dysfunctions and is typical of urge incontinence patients. An endurance index can be elaborated.

Squeezing: the maneuver by which the patient squeezes the anal sphincter as strongly as he can and maintains it. Squeezing maneuver must be performed by the patient for at least 20 s (not more than 30 s). In most protocols it is repeated three times letting patient to rest some seconds between different phases.

Thermal or pressure drift: the solid state sensors are susceptible to "thermal drift," that is, a change in measured pressure due to a change in temperature. With prolonged (1–2 h) studies, the baseline pressure drift over time appears to be linear. Thermal compensation is applied to the data during computerized analysis to compensate for this baseline drift [23].

Wave, Slow: waves with rhythmic activity, with frequency between 9 and 20 cycle\min, with variable width between 2 and 20 mmHg [24–26].

Wave, Ultraslow: waves with frequency between 0.5 and 1.5 cycle\min (they can be considered marker of severity in case of anal fissures and could have negative predictive value of the response to medical therapy with calcium blockers or nitric oxide donors drugs) [24].

References

1. Ambartsumyan L, Rodriguez L, Morera C, Nurko S. Longitudinal and radial characteristics of intra-anal pressures in children using 3D high-definition anorectal manometry: new observations. Am J Gastroenterol. 2013;108(12):1918–28.
2. Bordeianou LG, Carmichael JC, Paquette IM, Wexner S, Hull TL, Bernstein M, Keller DS, Zutshi M, Varma MG, Gurland BH, Steele SR. Consensus statement of definitions for anorectal physiology testing and pelvic floor terminology (revised). Dis Colon Rectum. 2018;61(4):421–7.
3. Coss-Adame E, Rao SS, Valestin J, Ali-Azamar A, Remes-Troche JM. Accuracy and reproducibility of high-definition anorectal manometry and pressure topography analyses in healthy subjects. Clin Gastroenterol Hepatol. 2015;13(6):1143–50.
4. Lee TH, Bharucha AE. How to perform and interpret a high-resolution anorectal manometry test. J Neurogastroenterol Motil. 2016;22(1):46–59.
5. Wu JF, Lu CH, Yang CH, Tsai IJ. Diagnostic role of anal sphincter relaxation integral in high-resolution anorectal manometry for hirschsprung disease in infants. J Pediatr. 2018;194:136–41.
6. Ratuapli S, Bharucha AE, Harvey D, Zinsmeister AR. Comparison of rectal balloon expulsion test in seated and left lateral positions. Neurogastroenterol Motil. 2013;25(12):e813–20.
7. Li Y, Yang X, Xu C, Zhang Y, Zhang X. Normal values and pressure morphology for three-dimensional high-resolution anorectal manometry of asymptomatic adults: a study in 110 subjects. Int J Color Dis. 2013;28(8):1161–8.
8. Bove A, Pucciani F, Bellini M, Battaglia E, Bocchini R, Altomare DF, Dodi G, Sciaudone G, Falletto E, Piloni V, Gambaccini D, Bove V. Consensus statement AIGO/SICCR: diagnosis and treatment of chronic constipation and obstructed defecation (part I: diagnosis). World J Gastroenterol. 2012;18(14):1555–64.
9. Chiarioni G, Kim SM, Vantini I, Whitehead WE. Validation of the balloon evacuation test: reproducibility and agreement with findings from anorectal manometry and electromyography. Clin Gastroenterol Hepatol. 2014;12(12):2049–54.
10. Ihnat P, Vavra P, Gunkova P, Pelikan A, Zonca P. 3D high resolution anorectal manometry in functional anorectal evaluation. Rozhl Chir. 2014;93(11):524–9.
11. Seong MK. Assessment of functional defecation disorders using anorectal manometry. Ann Surg Treat Res. 2018;94(6):330–6.
12. Seo M, Joo S, Jung KW, Lee J, Lee HJ, Soh JS, Yoon IJ, Koo HS, Seo SY, Kim D, Hwang SW, Park SH, Yang DH, Ye BD, Byeon JS, Jung HY, Yang SK, Rao SS, Myung SJ. A high-resolution anorectal manometry parameter based on integrated pressurized volume: a study based on 204 male patients with constipation and 26 controls. Neurogastroenterol Motil. 2018;30(9):e13376.
13. Grossi U, Carrington EV, Bharucha AE, Horrocks EJ, Scott SM, Knowles CH. Diagnostic accuracy study of anorectal manometry for diagnosis of dyssynergic defecation. Gut. 2016;65(3):447–55.
14. Rao SS, Bharucha AE, Chiarioni G, Felt-Bersma RJ, Knowles C, Malcolm A, Wald A. Functional anorectal disorders. Gastroenterology. 2016;150(6):1430–42.
15. Heinrich H, Misselwitz B. High-resolution anorectal manometry - new insights in the diagnostic assessment of functional anorectal disorders. Visc Med. 2018;34(2):134–9.
16. Dinning PG, Carrington EV, Scott SM. The use of colonic and anorectal high-resolution manometry and its place in clinical work and in research. Neurogastroenterol Motil. 2015;27(12):1693–708.
17. Viebig RG, Franco JTY, Araujo SV, Gualberto D. Water-perfused high-resolution anorectal manometry (HRAM-WP): the first Brazilian study. Arq Gastroenterol. 2018;55Suppl 1(Suppl 1):41–6.
18. Jung KW, Joo S, Yang DH, Yoon IJ, Seo SY, Kim SO, Lee J, Lee HJ, Kim KJ, Ye BD, Byeon JS, Jung HY, Yang SK, Kim JH, Myung SJ. A novel high-resolution anorectal manometry parameter based on a three-dimensional integrated pressurized volume of a spatiotemporal

plot, for predicting balloon expulsion in asymptomatic normal individuals. Neurogastroenterol Motil. 2014;26(7):937–49.

19. Seo M, Joo S, Jung KW, Song EM, Rao SSC, Myung SJ. New metrics in high-resolution and high-definition anorectal manometry. Curr Gastroenterol Rep. 2018;20(12):57.

20. Bajwa A, Thiruppathy K, Emmanuel A. The utility of conditioning sequences in barostat protocols for the measurement of rectal compliance. Color Dis. 2013;15(6):715–8.

21. Cheeney G, Nguyen M, Valestin J, Rao SS. Topographic and manometric characterization of the recto-anal inhibitory reflex. Neurogastroenterol Motil. 2012;24(3):e147–54.

22. Chedid V, Vijayvargiya P, Halawi H, Park SY, Camilleri M. Audit of the diagnosis of rectal evacuation disorders in chronic constipation. Neurogastroenterol Motil. 2019;31(1):e13510.

23. Parthasarathy G, McMaster J, Feuerhak K, Zinsmeister AR, Bharucha AE. Determinants and clinical impact of pressure drift in manoscan anorectal high resolution manometry system. Neurogastroenterol Motil. 2016;28(9):1433–7.

24. Opazo A, Aguirre E, Saldana E, Fantova MJ, Clave P. Patterns of impaired internal anal sphincter activity in patients with anal fissure. Color Dis. 2013;15(4):492–9.

25. Yoshino H, Kayaba H, Hebiguchi T, Morii M, Hebiguchi T, Itoh W, Chihara J, Kato T. Anal ultraslow waves and high anal pressure in childhood: a clinical condition mimicking Hirschsprung disease. J Pediatr Surg. 2007;42(8):1422–8.

26. Yoshino H, Kayaba H, Hebiguchi T, Morii M, Hebiguchi T, Ito W, Chihara J, Kato T. Multiple clinical presentations of anal ultra slow waves and high anal pressure: megacolon, hemorrhoids and constipation. Tohoku J Exp Med. 2007;211(2):127–32.

Correction to: Performing, Analyzing, and Interpreting HRAM and HDAM Recordings

Edda Battaglia, Lucia D'Alba, Antonella La Brocca, and Francesco Torresan

Correction to: M. Bellini (ed.), *High Resolution and High Definition Anorectal Manometry*, https://doi.org/10.1007/978-3-030-32679-1_7

The chapter "Performing, Analyzing, and Interpreting HRAM and HDAM Recordings" was inadvertently published without the reference and its citation within the text. The corrected version is available on doi: https://doi.org/10.1007/978-3-030-32419-3_11 with reference number 25.

The updated online version of this chapter can be found at https://doi.org/10.1007/978-3-030-32679-1_7